W9-CPD-874

Unlocking
Nature's Pharmacy™

www.unlockingnaturespharmacy.com

"One's mind, once stretched by a new idea, never regains it's original dimensions."

Oliver Wendel Holmes, M.D.
(1809-1894)**

**Dr. Holmes lived his life between the poetic and the realistic. A celebrated poet-doctor, he spent the greater part of his life as physician and professor at Harvard University teaching anatomy and physiology.

Unlocking
Nature's Pharmacy™

Mayer Eisenstein, M.D., J.D., M.P.H.

Published by CMI Press
http://www.unlockingnaturespharmacy.com

ISBN 0-9670444-99

$16.95

Printed in the United States of America

Books by Mayer Eisenstein, MD, JD, MPH

Home Birth Advantage

Safer Medicine

Don't Vaccinate Before You Educate

Unavoidably Dangerous (Medical Hazards of Synthetic Hormone Replacement Therapy)

Available at www.unlocking naturespharmacy.com

MEDICAL DISCLAIMER

Unlocking Nature's Pharmacy™ contains the opinions, based on scientific fact and evidence, of its author, Mayer Eisenstein, MD, JD, MPH. It is not intended to replace the advice of your physician or healthcare provider. If any reader requires personal medical attention, a competent medical professional should be consulted. The author and publisher disclaim any responsibility for any liability, loss or risk, personal or otherwise, which is incurred as a consequence, directly or indirectly, by the use and application of any of the contents of this book.

Table of Contents:

ACKNOWLEDGMENT

It is one thing to have an idea and quite another to turn that idea into reality. The following people have helped me turn many ideas into reality.

I am proud, honored and grateful to have worked with Drs. Peter Rosi, Paul Schattauer and Mark Zumhagen for over 20 years. I admire their dedication to the practice of scientific evidence based medicine. They truly exemplify physicians who abide by the Hippocratic Oath and for them nature's pharmacy has always been unlocked.

Lynne Klauss has been a vital part of our administration for the past 17 years. She has taken on many different tasks and been a wonderful liaison between our patients and staff. Her tireless effort and devotion to our medical practice is boundless and much appreciated.

For over 25 years I have been privileged to work with Fran Levitansky. Her continual help as my editor, patience with my many revisions, and willingness to be available for a myriad of seemingly endless projects have made her an invaluable asset to myself and my entire medical staff.

Dedication

In the spring of 2004, I helped a family successfully give birth at home. In the process I strained my back and continued to have difficulty walking for the next several weeks. I tried all types of remedies to no avail, including chiropractic care, even resorting to pharmaceutical drugs. My dear friend, Mark Mandel, compounding pharmacist and co-host of our weekly radio show "The Doctor and the Pharmacist" called me and said "Mayer, I want you to try this natural product." I told Mark that it probably would not work, but I would try it anyway. Within two weeks my back pain was gone and I was totally able to function. Subsequently, with the help of Mark Mandel, I formulated *AllFlex*™, a natural pharmaceutical to relieve muscle and joint pain.

Mark is a compounding pharmacist, with one of the most unique pharmacies in the Chicagoland area. Mark Drugs Pharmacy sells more natural products than pharmaceuticals. Whenever I, or one of my Homefirst® staff, need a remedy, my answer is always the same, "Call Mark". It is with great pleasure and honor that I dedicate *Unlocking Nature's Pharmacy*™ to my dear friend, co-host of our radio show, "The Doctor and The Pharmacist", Mark Mandel, without whom I would not have been inspired to add natural pharmaceuticals to my medical practice or to write this book.

Foreword

Mark H. Mandel R.Ph.

Humankind did not develop in a void. We grew into our world amongst plants and other animals. Many of the things that we typically consider unique about our species are actually shared by these plants and animals. Earliest man recognized this and used nature to improve the quality of life. Some plants were used to treat illness, other plants were used to enhance sensation or lessen pain. As man moved through the wilderness he would eat what he could collect or capture. Through these experiences - some good and some lethal – he learned that different animal or plant parts could give him more energy and traditions developed such as eating a particular animal body part before going into battle. Some of these were symbolic but others were based on legitimate responses of the body.

In virtually all cultures there developed an individual or groups of individuals known as medicine men or healers. These earliest healers were physician, pharmacist and frequently clergy all built into one. They used a combination of plants, animals, minerals and faith to treat and cure illness or disease. As time progressed, the body of knowledge grew and these healers became more proficient in their disciplines. They started to specialize and although this focus allowed them to become progressively more adept and knowledgeable within their specialty, their ability to treat the 'whole' individual was progressively lost.

In the early part of the 20th century, western culture discovered antibiotics. It is interesting that these were not initially created in a laboratory but were discovered from a natural source, i.e. mold. The discovery of antibiotics was a landmark change in modern western medicine. Prior to this, healers could only ameliorate illness or disease, not cure it. The success of this new class of prepared drug treatment, which treats only infection, overshadows the significance of much that had been used before. This overshadowing crossed over into virtually all aspects of western healthcare and medicine bought into the idea that since manufactured antibiotics could 'cure' a condition then other manufactured drugs should be able to 'cure' other conditions. As a result of this surge in manufactured medication prominence the use of natural and herbal products was largely disregarded. These natural products were no less effective than they had been previously, but the words "new and improved" could not be used to market them.

By the mid-1960's, the use of drugs designed and prepared by manufacturers controlled the prescription market in the United States. Many clinicians in Europe continued to use homeopathy and herbal medicine. Eastern (Oriental) practitioners used herbs as their cornerstone of treatment but physicians in the U.S. and Canada who preferred herbal and natural treatments were largely discredited and considered oddities.

Many manufactured drugs are similar to products that occur in nature. This makes sense since drugs are designed to have a physiologic effect and many of these advanced, aggressive drugs have their origins in naturally occurring substances. Why, you may ask, do we simply not use the naturally occurring drugs that nature provides? The answer is simple: there's no money in it! Products that occur in nature cannot be patented. The huge profits that are associated with a patent, that can be protected, are what drive the multi-billion dollar pharmaceutical industry.

I have tremendous respect for the medical community and for physicians in general. These are typically people who are both brilliant and compassionate and who entered their respective fields with the intention of doing good and of making a difference in people's lives. Unfortunately, we can all fall prey to pressures around us. These pressures may be social, professional or our own fear of failure. As professionals who are perpetually short on time and who are expected to always have the right answers, it is sometimes simply easier to repeat the answers that are popularly accepted rather than look beyond at alternative solutions.

I started pharmacy school with a chip on my shoulder. When I was an under-graduate student I was injured in an accident. All the doctors would do was give me medicine for pain and muscle spasms. They never seemed to look for the source of the pain or offer other options for coping or improving the condition. Ironically, it was a pharmacist who explained to me that prescription drugs were not the answer. He convinced me to look at alternatives. This was my start to searching for the best answers to patient care and again ironically what prompted me to become a pharmacist. I no longer believed that all the medical answers could be found through prescription medications. I started to look at exercise, stretching, meditation, diet, herbs, salves and a variety of other alternative treatments for pain. Soon I discovered that there was a whole world out there besides that of traditional western medicine.

This approach soon led me to look at alternative treatments for other maladies and conditions. Granted, there are times that western medicine is effective and necessary, but there are many times that we miss the forest for the trees and fail to look for a cause of a problem or an alternative, less invasive approach to treatment. Western medicine is wonderful in that it is very fast and aggressive, but a fast easy fix that gets a patient over the hump isn't always the best or even only solution for the long term. Quite often the fast, easy, aggressive drug treatment is burdened with aggressive side effects.

Treatment of chronic conditions such as hypertension, dyslipidemia, thyroid imbalance, insulin resistance, diabetes, hormonal imbalance or even chronic pain may be better controlled with lifestyle changes including dietary modifications, exercise and supplementation than with drugs alone. All of these chronic conditions are influenced by the world around us and will frequently respond to treatments other than those of prescription medications.

There are a plethora of products on the market that offer to solve all the ills of mankind. Unfortunately there is not a single easily accessible source of information that tells which products actually work and how well they work. Nor is there a reliable source of information that tells which brands or combinations of products are potent and effective. There have been studies by independent researchers that have shown various classes of supplements to have less than 10% of the active ingredients that the products claimed to contain. In addition there are no real guidelines or dictates that are required of the nutritional, health food or supplement industries regarding testing, manufacturing processes or potency of ingredients contained in these products.

This lack of product requirements and support is troubling not only to consumers of these products but also to practitioners who wish to recommend or order these potentially very useful products to their patients and clients. Proper storage of products is typically inadequately described to retailers or consumers. As a result it is difficult to make an informed decision regarding which products to use and when to use them. It is therefore necessary to trust someone who is able to filter out products that do not meet certain standards of potency and purity. Although there are no legally mandated requirements for these products, that does not mean that there are not known requirements for the content and efficacy of these products.

Clarity and explanation of risks, benefits, positives and negatives are necessary for consumers to be guided in their allopathic and their alternative healthcare choices. That is what this book tries to do. It is an attempt to provide the consumer as well as the healthcare professional with a primer, an initial guide to the use of natural products that may be used to enhance life and improve health. Granted, there is no complete substitute for an able and informed healthcare practitioner. Whether that person is a pharmacist, physician, licensed dietitian or nutritionist is inconsequential. It is necessary that someone is present to hold herbal and nutritional manufacturers accountable just as it is necessary for government agencies to hold pharmaceutical manufacturers accountable for their products. As consumers, we need someone who can ask the proper questions and demand the appropriate answers. Otherwise, how do any of us know what we are actually getting?

The conditions that are described in this book are those chronic conditions that have been identified by virtually all healthcare organizations, private and public, as disorders that have a negative impact on both morbidity and mortality. There are many exceptional herbal and nutritional products on the market. In this book specific products are periodically recommended. It must be noted that there is no product that is universally appropriate for every person and every condition but there are certain guidelines that should be followed when devising a course of treatment. Dr. Eisenstein has followed those guidelines and has presented a roadmap. Just like any roadmap, there are alternative pathways that may be followed. Different excursions will provide different experiences but hopefully this roadmap will guide you, the consumer towards better health while using some of the tools and treatments that nature has afforded us.

Introduction

Natural vs. Synthetic Pharmaceuticals

(There will be many new words introduced throughout this text, we encourage you to refer to the "Glossary" which we have made as comprehensive as possible.)

Chronic illness, such as high blood pressure, high cholesterol, muscle and joint pain, arthritis, allergy, chronic fatigue syndrome and asthma are not just the province of the elderly. How common are chronic illnesses? In a study published in the *Annals of Family Medicine* May-June 2005, 980 adults were treated by 21 family doctors, 9 out of 10 patients had more than one chronic condition, and nearly half of the middle aged patients (45-64) had five or more chronic conditions. The most common illnesses were high blood pressure, high cholesterol, and muscle and joint pain. What do these numbers have to do with you? An estimated 57,000,000 people were diagnosed with multiple chronic conditions in 2000 and that number is expected to reach 81,000,000 by 2020.

The pharmaceutical companies that create synthetic drugs are brilliant. Their blood pressure, cholesterol, muscle and joint pain drugs have increased our life span, but have they comprised our quality of life? A study in the January 2006 issue of the *Journal of the American Geriatrics Society* found that simvastatin [Zocor® and the entire family of statins Lipitor®, Crestor®, Prevacor®, etc.] "has statistically significant effects on affect and affective processes in elderly volunteers. The decrease in positive affect may be significant clinically and relevant to the quality of life of many patients."

The problem is that the compounds that they create to control blood pressure, cholesterol and muscle and joint pain are not completely natural in their biochemical profile. It is not that the body cannot digest these compounds, but they put more stress on the liver and kidneys than substances found in nature. In order to patent their designer synthetic drugs, the pharmaceutical companies must alter the natural chemical structure. These altered synthetic chemicals have been linked to many serious side-effects. The family of statin drugs, which has been shown to lower cholesterol levels, has side effects which include abdominal pain, allergic reactions, back pain, changes in eyesight, constipation, diarrhea, dry eyes, dry skin, hair loss, headache, heartburn, leg cramps, muscle aching or weakness, neuromuscular degeneration, transient memory loss (read about this at www.spacedoc.net) and in rare situations rhabdomyolysis (a muscle condition that can cause kidney failure). The family of high blood pressure medications (beta blockers, ace inhibitors, calcium channel blockers, diuretics, etc.) has side effects which include: dry mouth, headache, dizziness, vomiting, fatigue, depression, GI upset, diarrhea, low pulse, sexual dysfunction to name just a few. The family of muscle and joint pain medications (Vioxx®, Bextra®, Celebrex®, Mobid®, NSAIDS, aspirin, Tylenol®), has side effects which include: fever, sneezing, chest congestion, cough, sore throat, swelling in the arms and legs, trouble sleeping, dizziness, lack of appetite, diarrhea, difficulty breathing, yellowing of the skin, eye problems, sluggishness, fatigue, unexplained weight gain, heart attacks, etc.

Why natural products? Whenever we start with a natural molecule, we are building on substances which nature has refined over thousands of years. These substances can be digested and metabolized by our enzymes, liver and kidneys without any serious side effects. When we ingest synthetic substances our organ systems do not have the proper digestive enzymes to completely metabolize them, thus leading to many of the side effects we suffer from.

Everyone agrees that lowering blood pressure, lowering cholesterol and relief from muscle and joint pain are desirable. It would be nice if we had natural products with minimal side effects which could produce the same effects of lowering blood pressure, lowering cholesterol level and reducing muscle and joint pain. Thankfully these natural products do exist and can be used successfully, sometimes in conjunction with synthetic pharmaceuticals, but many times on their own. My goal here is not to tell you not to use synthetic pharmaceuticals when necessary, but when feasible to replace them with natural pharmaceuticals.

You may have high blood pressure and high cholesterol levels and not be aware of it. These parameters can be documented by physical measurements, i.e. blood pressure cuff, stethoscope and blood test. Therefore, it is easy to assess if the natural pharmaceuticals that you are taking are lowering your blood pressure and cholesterol levels. As part of a healthy program, along with good diet, exercise and healthy lifestyle, I recommend that you see your doctor to assure that the natural pharmaceuticals are having the desired effect.

As pathogenic bacteria become resistant to antibiotics, scientists are looking to other means to combat infections. We are seeing just the infancy in the use of probiotics and prebiotics, both for health maintenance and for treating different medical conditions. Probiotics are the live friendly bacteria or live friendly yeast that we can take as natural pharmaceuticals. As the scientific literature documents, probiotics have a protective effect against allergy, eczema, infection, diarrhea, blood pressure, cholesterol and more. Prebiotics are non-digestible food ingredients that beneficially affect the host by selectively stimulating the growth of one or a more friendly bacteria in the colon.

I recommend that you find a doctor who understands and prescribes, when feasible, natural pharmaceuticals for health maintenance, as well as alternatives to traditional blood pressure, cholesterol, muscle and joint pain medications, antibiotics and other drug pharmaceuticals.

Hippocrates, the father of modern medicine, said that the order of health is first-regimen, second-medicine and last-surgery. Regimen, according to Hippocrates, consisted of lifestyle, diet, exercise, etc. Only after you exhaust different facets of regimen, do you move onto medicine and only after you exhaust medicine do you move onto surgery. In this country we do things backwards. First we do surgery, if that fails we use medicine and if medicine fails we go to regimen. Only after surgery and medicine fail do we look towards alternative treatments. Following Hippocrates advice let us use regimen first, medicine secondarily and surgery only as a last resort.

My goal is to introduce you to the world of natural pharmaceuticals and as such increase your quality as well as quantity of life. Use all of the available resources: books, internet, pharmacists and medical practitioners to learn more about natural pharmaceuticals.

Mayer Eisenstein, MD, JD, MPH

Primum Non Nocere (Above all do no harm)

Hippocrates, circa 460BC**

Hippocratic Oath

" I swear by Apollo the physician, by Aesculapius, Hygeia, and Panacea, and I take to witness all the gods, and all the goddesses, to keep according to my ability and my judgment the following Oath: To consider dear to me as my parents him who taught me this art; to live in common with him and if necessary to share my goods with him; to look upon his children as my own brothers, to teach them this art if they so desire without fee or written promise; to impart to my sons and the sons of the master who taught me and disciples who have enrolled themselves and have agreed to the rules of the profession, but to these alone, the precepts and the instruction. I will prescribe regimen for the good of my patients according to my ability and by judgement and never do harm to anyone. To please no one will I prescribe a deadly drug, nor give advice which may cause his death. Nor will I give a woman a pessary to procure abortion. But I will preserve the purity of my life and my art. I will not cut for stone, even for patients in whom the disease is manifest; I will leave this operation to be performed by practitioners (specialists in this art). In every house where I come I will enter only for the good of my patients, keeping myself far from all intentional ill-doing and all seduction, and especially from the pleasures of love with women or with men, be they free or slaves. All that may come to my knowledge in the exercise of my profession or outside of my profession or in daily commerce with men, which ought not to be spread abroad, I will keep secret and will never reveal. If I keep this oath faithfully, may I enjoy my life and practice my art, respected by all men and in all times; but if I swerve from it or violate it, may the reverse be my lot."

ME COMMENTS:

We must remind doctors of the oath of Hippocrates which they took upon graduating from medical school, "Primum Non Nocere" - Above All Do No Harm.

***A statement, attributed to the ancient Greek physician Hippocrates, the father of modern medicine, that serves as an ethical guide for physicians and is incorporated into the graduation ceremonies at many medical schools. The duties "to do no harm" and of confidentiality are based in the Hippocratic oath.*

Preface

Synergistic Effect

There are many studies on the beneficial effects of different natural pharmaceuticals for various medical conditions. However, there are few studies concerning the synergistic effect of combining different natural products. I am looking forward to using the scientific literature to combine various natural products which will work on various chronic medical conditions.

The combined products can be more effective than individual ones, easier to take (less capsules or pills) and less expensive than the individual ingredients separately. Please refer to my web page www.unlockingnaturespharmacy.com.

BLOOD PRESSURE

Hypertension is a serious medical problem that has been linked to an increased risk of heart attack and stroke. Recent scientific studies have shown that over 50% of Americans over the age of 40 have either elevated blood pressure or elevated cholesterol levels. A newly defined condition **"prehypertension"** (systolic 121-139 / diastolic 81-89) has been shown to increase risk of heart attack and coronary vessel disease (CVD). Prehypertension presents a dilemma for the treating physician. This condition should not be ignored, it should be treated beyond diet, exercise and lifestyle. Natural pharmaceuticals, prescribed at this early stage could help prevent these "warning signs" from becoming life-threatening problems.

Scientific literature shows that pharmaceuticals, (i.e. beta blockers, ace inhibitors, calcium channel blockers, diuretics, etc.) can lower blood pressure. However, these medications have side effects which make compliance difficult. Dry mouth, headache, dizziness, vomiting, fatigue, depression, GI upset, diarrhea, slow pulse, sexual dysfunction are just a sampling of the side effects that cause patients to stray from following their doctors recommendations.

Bonito Peptides, Omega 3 Fish Oil, CoezymeQ10, Folic Acid, Stevia and Probiotics especially Lactobacillus Helveticus are natural products which have been scientifically demonstrated to lower blood pressure without any type of side effects.

Bonito peptides are a natural product derived from the Bonito fish. The peptides are extracted, purified and independently assayed for heavy metals, pesticides and other contaminants. These peptides have ace inhibitor activity which lowers blood pressure. They exert their effect by inhibiting the angiotensin converting enzyme (ace) which causes blood pressure to go up. They can successfully reduce blood pressure in a large percentage of people without additional use of pharmaceuticals. There have been no reported side effects from bonito peptides.

Lactobacillus helveticus, has been shown to lower blood pressure. My suspicion is that it acts like a natural ace inhibitor, as we know that all lactobacilli have some ace inhibitor activity.

Stevia is an herb with incredible sweetening power. Its ability to sweeten is rated between 70 and 400 times that of white sugar. It is completely natural in its biochemical profile. Unlike other natural sweetening agents, it is completely calorie free; never initiates a rise in blood sugar, does not provide food for microorganisms like bacteria and yeast, and has been shown to lower blood pressure.

Omega3 Fatty Acids are composed of polyunsaturated fatty acids which are found mainly in fish such as tuna and salmon, fish oils, green leafy vegetables, and some vegetable oils. A diet rich in Omega 3 has been shown to lower cholesterol and blood pressure levels. The American Heart Association recommends Omega3 fish oils either from the actual fish (tuna, salmon, etc.) or from natural supplements.

The synergistic effect of adding two or more natural pharmaceuticals together may be the next step in maintaining health, as well as treating a disease processes.

CoenzymeQ10 (or *ubiquinone*) is a cofactor in the mitochondrial electron transport chain, the biochemical pathway in cellular respiration from which adenosine triphosphate (ATP) and metabolic energy are derived. Since nearly all cellular activities are dependent upon energy, Coenzyme Q10 is essential for the health of all human tissues and organs.

Coenzyme Q10 is a naturally occurring antioxidant nutrient which retards free radical formation in biological systems. Coenzyme Q10 resembles vitamin E and vitamin K in chemical structure. Biochemically, it functions much like vitamin E in that it participates in antioxidant and free radical reactions. Healthy persons who consume a well balanced diet, one high in vitamins, minerals, and other nutrient factors, have the ability to synthesize Coenzyme Q10. Unhealthy individuals and those eating an inadequate diet may not synthesize Coenzyme Q10 in sufficient quantity. It has been shown that in disease states, nutrients from food sources may not necessarily be absorbed or available. Humans can biosynthesize Coenzyme Q10 from tyrosine or phenylalanine and mevalonic acid. This complex biochemical process requires 15 separate steps and many enzymes, coenzymes, vitamins and minerals. Only by such a process can the respiratory chain receive proper levels of Coenzyme Q10.

Scientific studies indicate Coenzyme Q10 also plays an important role in the maintenance of the entire cardiovascular system. Supplementation with Coenzyme Q10 in patients has been shown to be useful in the maintenance of healthy blood pressure. For people taking statin drugs, supplementation with CoQ10 is especially important, since all statins interfere with the pathway leading to production of CoQ10.

Folic acid is essential for the synthesis of adenine and thymine, two of the four nucleic acids that make up our genes, DNA and chromosomes. It is also required for the proper metabolism of the essential amino acid methionine that is found primarily in animal proteins. A folic acid deficiency has been linked to an elevated level of homocysteine, a sulfur-containing amino acid. High homocysteine levels, in turn, have been linked to cardiovascular disease and a host of other unhealthy conditions.

Research by Dr. Jeremiah Stamler, a scientist who has devoted his whole life to the researching of hypertension, demonstrated in a 1996 study that there was an inverse relationship between dietary protein and blood pressure (i.e. higher protein in the diet resulted in a lower blood pressure). The late Dr. Robert Atkins, cardiologist, in his life work on diet, also showed that high protein in the diet also lowered blood pressure and cholesterol levels. It is interesting that the most effective natural pharmaceutical to have an effect on blood pressure is the bonito peptides. It seems that many diverse scientific studies lead to the same conclusion: lower refined sugars and higher protein diets lower blood pressure and cholesterol levels.

It is important to monitor the blood pressure to be sure that the natural pharmaceutical alternatives are exerting the proper blood pressure lowering effect. Preliminary data has shown that over 70% of people can either reduce or terminate use of pharmaceutical medication by using these natural substitutes.

It may take some time to find the right combination of natural pharmaceuticals to lower your blood pressure. It is important to remember that the goal is to lower the blood pressure. If the natural pharmaceuticals are not bringing about this result you must consider using drug pharmaceuticals or a combination of the two.

The following scientific studies document the evidence based approach to using various natural pharmaceuticals that may lower your blood pressure levels.

ଔଓଔଓ

Hypertension & Life Expectancy

In the journal *Hypertension* (2005;46:280.)

Dr. Oscar H. Franco, et al. studied

"Blood Pressure in Adulthood and Life Expectancy With Cardiovascular Disease in Men and Women"

Conclusion: "Irrespective of sex, 50-year-old hypertensives compared with normotensives had a shorter life expectancy, a shorter life expectancy free of cardiovascular disease, myocardial infarction, and stroke, and a longer life expectancy lived with these diseases. Normotensive men (22% of men) survived 7.2 years (95% confidence interval, 5.6 to 9.0) longer without cardiovascular disease compared with hypertensives and spent 2.1 (0.9 to 3.4) fewer years of life with cardiovascular disease. Similar differences were observed in women. **Compared with hypertensives, total life expectancy was 5.1 and 4.9 years longer for normotensive men and women, respectively.** Increased blood pressure in adulthood is associated with large reductions in life expectancy and more years lived with cardiovascular disease. This effect is larger than estimated previously and affects both sexes similarly. Our findings underline the tremendous importance of preventing high blood pressure and its consequences in the population."

ME COMMENT:

How much would we give to increase our life expectancy? This is one study that actually quantifies in years the effect of normal vs. high blood pressure. 5.1 years for men and 4.9 years for women.

ଓଷଓଷ

Prehypertension

In the journal *Annals of Family Medicine* 3:294-299 (2005)

Dr. Heather A. Liszka, et al. studied

"Prehypertension and Cardiovascular Morbidity"

PURPOSE: The Seventh Report of the Joint National Commission (JNC 7) on High Blood Pressure established prehypertension (120 to 139 mm Hg systolic or 80 to 89 mm Hg diastolic) as a new risk category. We aim to determine the risk of major cardiovascular events associated with blood pressure in the prehypertensive range in a longitudinal, population-based cohort...

CONCLUSIONS: In a longitudinal, population-based, US cohort, prehypertension was associated with increased risk of major cardiovascular events independently of other cardiovascular risk factors. These findings, along with the presence of cardiovascular risk factors in the majority of participant sample with prehypertension, support recommendations for physicians to actively target lifestyle modifications and multiple risk reduction in their prehypertensive patients.

ME COMMENTS:

Prehypertension is a real risk factor for heart attack and CAD. Even though there is no recommendation to use pharmaceuticals at this time, I would recommend using natural pharmaceuticals for this condition.

ঙ্কঙ্ক

Prehypertension

In the journal *Stroke* (2005;36:1859.)

Dr. Adnan I. Qureshi, et al. studied

"Is Prehypertension a Risk Factor for Cardiovascular Diseases?"

Background and Purpose— The Joint National Committee on High Blood Pressure identified a new category of blood pressure in adults termed prehypertension. Our objective was to determine the long- term risk of cardiovascular diseases associated with this new category in a well-defined cohort of adults.

Methods— We evaluated the association of prehypertension (120 to 139/80 to 89 mm Hg) and hypertension (>140/90 mm Hg) with the incidence of atherothrombotic brain infarction (ABI), all strokes, myocardial infarction (MI), and coronary artery disease (CAD)...

Conclusions— Prehypertension appears to be associated with an increased risk of MI and CAD but not stroke. Further studies are required to confirm the anticipated benefits of identifying and intervening in persons with pre-hypertension.

ME COMMENTS:

Dr. Qureshi found that, unlike high blood pressure, prehypertension is linked to a higher risk of heart attack and coronary artery disease but not stroke. Dr. Qureshi struggles with the treatment plan for prehypertension. He states: "while we classically recommend lifestyle modification, such as weight control, regular physical activity, and changes in diet for people with prehypertension, these findings (the above study) raise the question of whether we should treat pre-hypertensive patients more aggressively." There is a very simple solution for prehypertension regimen: diet, exercise, weight control and natural pharmaceuticals.

ଓଃ ଓଃ

Protein in Diet

In the journal *Circulation* (1996;94:1629-1634.)

Dr. J. Stamler, MD, et al., studied...

"Inverse Relation of Dietary Protein Markers With Blood Pressure

Findings for 10,020 Men and Women in the INTERSALT Study"

The purpose of this study was to assess relations to blood pressure (BP) in individuals of markers of dietary protein in their 24-hour urine collections....

...that higher dietary protein intake has favorable influences on BP.

ME COMMENTS:

Dr. Stamler, a recognized expert in the field of hypertension, cholesterol and diabetes has been a long time advocate of low fat diets. This study points out that a high protein diet may be one of the answers for hypertension. The government food pyramid is changing from a high carbohydrate and low protein diet to a slightly higher protein, slightly lower carbohydrate diet.

However, this is still missing the point! What the evidence proves is that high protein is one of the factors to lower your blood pressure.

To further prove the point that lowfat diets are not the answer, the February 2006 Journal of the AMA (JAMA), reported on an 8 year study (costing $415,000,000) which showed that eating less fat and increasing grain intake late in life failed to lower the risk of breast cancer, colon cancer and heart disease.

ଔଓଔଓ

Protein in Diet

In the journal *Hypertension.* 2001;38:821.

Valerie Burke, et al., studied

"Dietary Protein and Soluble Fiber Reduce Ambulatory Blood Pressure in Treated Hypertensives"

And found that...

...In the 36 subjects who provided complete data, protein and fiber had significant additive effects to lower 24-hour and awake systolic blood pressure. Relative to control subjects, the net reduction in 24-hour systolic blood pressure was 5.9 mm Hg with fiber and with protein. Findings were independent of age, gender, and change in weight, alcohol intake, or urinary sodium and potassium. Relative to reduced fiber and protein intake, dietary protein and soluble fiber supplements lower blood pressure additively in hypertensives. These findings have important implications for the prevention and management of hypertension, particularly in populations in which high blood pressure is prevalent in association with diets low in protein, fiber, or both.

ME COMMENTS:

This study points out that a diet which eliminates refined carbohydrates will lower blood pressure.

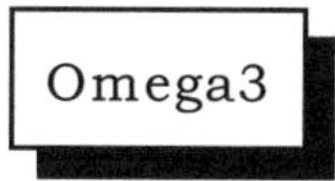

In the *Journal of the American College of Cardiology,* 2005; 46:120-124

Dr. Antonis Zampelas, et al., studied...

"Fish Consumption Among Healthy Adults Is Associated With Decreased Levels of Inflammatory Markers Related to Cardiovascular Disease"

CONCLUSIONS: Fish consumption,(especially fish rich in Omega 3 fatty acids, such as salmon, mackeral, and tuna, at least 10 oz. per week) was independently associated with lower inflammatory markers levels, among healthy adults. The strength and consistency of this finding has implications for public health and should be explored further.

ME COMMENTS:

Omega3 Fatty Acids seem to have a greater effect if they come from fish or fish supplements rather than from plant supplements.

ꕥꕥꕥꕥ

Lactobacillus Helveticus

American Journal of Clinical Nutrition, Vol. 77, No. 2, 326-330, February 2003

Seppo, Leena, et al., studied

"A fermented milk high in bioactive peptides has a blood pressure–lowering effect in hypertensive subjects"

Background: Angiotensin-converting enzyme (ACE; EC 3.4.15.1) plays a dual role in the regulation of hypertension: it catalyzes the production of the vasoconstrictor angiotensin II and it inactivates the vasodilator bradykinin. By inhibiting these processes, ACE inhibitors have antihypertensive effects. Peptides derived from milk proteins can have ACE-inhibiting properties and may thus be used as antihypertensive components.

Objective: We evaluated the long-term blood pressure–lowering effect of milk fermented by Lactobacillus helveticus LBK-16H in hypertensive subjects.

Design: In a randomized placebo-controlled study, 39 hypertensive patients received 150 mL/d of either L. helveticus LBK-16H fermented milk or a control product for 21 wk after a 2-wk run-in period. During the run-in period, the average baseline diastolic and systolic blood pressure values were 155 and 97 mm Hg, respectively, in the test product group and 152 and 96 mm Hg, respectively, in the control group. After the run-in period, blood pressure was measured at home on the same day every week with the use of an automatic blood pressure recorder.

Results: There was a mean difference of 6.7 ± 3.0 mm Hg in systolic blood pressure (P = 0.030) and of 3.6 ± 1.9 mm Hg (P = 0.059) in diastolic blood pressure between the test product and control groups. Demographic factors had no significant effect on the responses.

Conclusion: L. helveticus LBK-16H fermented milk containing bioactive peptides in normal daily use has a blood pressure–lowering effect in hypertensive subjects.

ME COMMENTS:

In Dr. Seepo's study lactobacillus helveticus lowered the systolic pressure by 6.7mm Hg and the diastolic pressure by 3.6 mm Hg. While this alone is not a major reduction, when used synergistically with other natural products shown to lower blood pressure, i.e. stevia, bonito peptides, folic acid, a major reduction can take place.

ꟹꟹ

Lactobacillus Helveticus

In the *American Journal of Clinical Nutrition.* 2005; 24(4):257-65

Dr. K. Aihara, et al., studied...

"Effect of powdered fermented milk with Lactobacillus helveticus on subjects with high-normal blood pressure or mild hypertension."

CONCLUSIONS: Daily ingestion of the tablets containing powdered fermented milk with L. helveticus CM4 in subjects with high-normal blood pressure or mild hypertension reduces elevated blood pressure without any adverse effects.

ME COMMENTS:

Evidence that the probiotic friendly bacteria, Lactobacillus helveticus, may be used to lower blood pressure.

ଔଋଔଋ

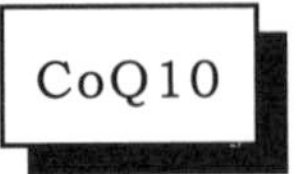

In the Journal *Biofactors* - 01-JAN-2003; 18(1-4): 91-100

F. Rosenfeldt, et al., studied...

"Systematic review of effect of coenzyme Q10 in physical exercise, hypertension and heart failure."

And found...

...We identified eight published trials of CoQ10 in hypertension. Altogether in the eight studies the mean decrease in systolic blood pressure was 16 mm Hg and in diastolic blood pressure, 10 mm Hg. Being devoid of significant side effects **CoQ10 may have a role as an adjunct or alternative to conventional agents in the treatment of hypertension....**

ଔଋଔଋ

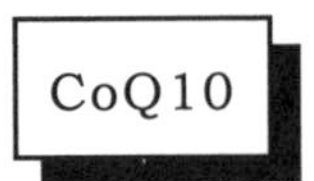

In the Journal *Biofactors* - 01-JAN-2003; 18(1-4): 129-36

JM Hodgson, et al. studied...

"Can Coenzyme Q10 improve vascular function and blood pressure? Potential for effective therapeutic reduction in vascular oxidative stress."

And found...

Coenzyme Q10 (CoQ) is an endogenously synthesised compound that acts as an electron carrier in the mitochondrial electron transport chain. The presence of adequate tissue concentrations of CoQ may be important in limiting oxidative and nitrosative damage in vivo. Oxidative and nitrosative stress are likely to be elevated in conditions such as diabetes and hypertension. In these conditions elevated oxidative and nitrosative stress within the arterial wall may contribute to increased blood pressure and vascular dysfunction. The major focus of this review is the potential of CoQ to improve vascular function and lower blood pressure. Although there is substantial indirect support for the putative mechanism of effect of CoQ on the vascular system, to date there is little direct support for an effect of CoQ on in vivo markers of oxidative or nitrosative stress. **The limited data available from studies in animal models and from human intervention studies are generally consistent with a benefit of CoQ on vascular function and blood pressure.** The observed effects of CoQ on these endpoints are potentially important therapeutically. However, before any firm clinical recommendations can be made about CoQ supplementation, further intervention studies in humans are needed to investigate the effects of CoQ on vascular function, blood pressure and cardiovascular outcomes. The particularly relevant groups of patients for these studies are those with insulin resistance, type 2 diabetes, hypertension and the metabolic syndrome.

ME COMMENTS:

If a drug pharmaceutical demonstrates any positive effect on blood pressure doctors embrace it automatically, even though they know that drug pharmaceuticals for high blood pressure have serious, and often unpleasant side effects. If a natural pharmaceutical, with no known side effects such as CoQ10, is found to lower blood pressure, instead of endorsing it doctors call for more studies.

ଔଔଔଔ

Bonito Peptides

In the journal *Comp Biochem Physiol C.* 1993 Feb;104(2):351-3.

H. Karaki et al studied...

"Oral administration of Peptides derived from Bonito bowels decreases blood pressure in spontaneously hypertensive rats by inhibiting angiotensin converting enzyme."

...Peptides... extracted from the autolysis product of Bonito liver and intestine, have been shown to inhibit angiotensin converting enzyme (ACE) activity in vitro... Oral administration of these Peptides... inhibited the pressor effect of intravenously administered angiotensin I in Sprague-Dawley rats. ...In spontaneously hypertensive rats, oral administration of these Peptides... showed depressor [lowering blood pressure] effects. ...**These results suggest that the Peptides... [they are referring to Bonito Peptides] are orally effective ACE inhibitors with hypotensive effect.**

ME COMMENTS:

Some of the best scientific research comes from veterinary medicine. Here Dr. Karaki demonstrates that bonito peptides lower blood pressure in rats by acting as an ACE inhibitor. The ACE inhibitors are a class of pharmaceuticals which lower blood pressure.

I have clinically experienced the same blood pressure lowering results with many of my patients who have elevated blood pressure.

ଓଡଓଡ

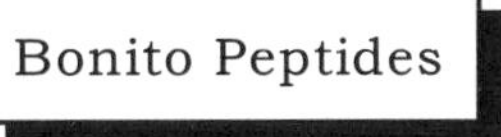

In the journal *Bioscience, Biotechnology and Biochemistry* 1993 Dec;57(12):2186-8.

M. Fujii, et al., studied...

"Antihypertensive effects of peptides in autolysate of bonito bowels on spontaneously hypertensive rats."

And found...

...Oral administration of the partially purified autolysate [the product of the breakdown of all or part of a cell or tissue by self-produced enzymes] decreased the systolic blood pressure of spontaneously hypertensive rats (SHR) in a dose-dependent manner at the doses of 1 g peptides/kg or higher.

ME COMMENTS:

In plain English, bonito peptides lowered blood pressure in hypertensive rats.

ଔଓଔଓ

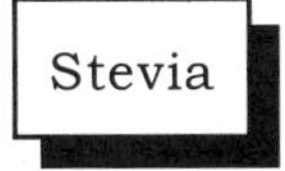

In the journal *Clinical Therapeutics*, 2003; 25(11):2797-808

MH Hsieh, et al., studied...

"Efficacy and tolerability of oral stevioside in patients with mild essential hypertension: a two-year, randomized, placebo-controlled study."

BACKGROUND: Stevioside, a natural glycoside isolated from the plant Stevia rebaudiana Bertoni, has been used as a commercial sweetening agent in Japan and Brazil for >20 years. Previous animal and human studies have indicated that stevioside has an antihypertensive effect. OBJECTIVES: This study was undertaken to investigate the long-term (2-year) efficacy and tolerability of stevioside in patients with mild essential hypertension. Secondary objectives were to determine the effects of stevioside on left ventricular mass index (LVMI) and quality of life (QOL). METHODS: This was a multicenter, randomized, double-blind, placebo-controlled trial in Chinese men and women aged between 20 and 75 years with mild essential hypertension (systolic blood pressure [SBP] 140-159 mm Hg and diastolic blood pressure [DBP] 90-99 mm Hg). Patients took capsules containing 500 mg stevioside powder or placebo 3 times daily for 2 years. Blood pressure was measured at monthly clinic visits; patients were also encouraged to monitor blood pressure at home using an automated device. RESULTS: One hundred seventy-four patients (87 men, 87 women) were enrolled in the study, and 168 completed it: 82 (42 men, 40 women; mean [SD] age, 52 years) in the stevioside group and 86 (44 women, 42 men; mean age, 53 years) in the placebo group. After 2 years, the stevioside group had significant decreases in mean (SD) SBP and DBP compared with baseline (SBP, from 150 [7.3] to 140 [6.8] mm Hg; DBP, from 95 [4.2] to 89 [3.2] mm Hg; $P < 0.05$) and compared with placebo ($P < 0.05$). Based on patients' records of self-monitored blood pressure, these effects were noted beginning approximately 1 week after the start of treatment and persisted throughout the study. There were no significant changes in body mass index or blood biochemistry, and the results of laboratory tests were similar in the 2 groups throughout the study....

...CONCLUSIONS: In this 2-year study in Chinese patients with mild hypertension, oral stevioside significantly decreased SBP [systolic blood pressure] and DBP [diastolic blood pressure] compared with placebo. QOL [quality of life] was improved, and no significant adverse effects were noted.

☙❧☙❧

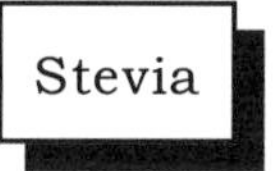

In the *British Journal of Clinical Pharmacology,* 2000; 50(3):215-20

P. Chan, et al., studied...

"A double-blind placebo-controlled study of the effectiveness and tolerability of oral stevioside in human hypertension."

AIMS: Stevioside is a natural plant glycoside isolated from the plant Stevia rebaudiana which has been commercialized as a sweetener in Japan for more than 20 years. Previous animal studies have shown that stevioside has an antihypertensive effect. This study was to designed to evaluate the effect of stevioside in human hypertension. METHODS: A multicentre, randomized, double-blind, placebo-controlled study was undertaken. This study group consisted of 106 Chinese hypertensive subjects with diastolic blood pressure between 95 and 110 mmHg and ages ranging from 28 to 75 years with 60 subjects (men 34, women 26; mean +/- s.d., 54.1+/-3.8 years) allocated to active treatment and 46 (men 19, women 27; mean +/- s.d., 53.7+/-4.1 years) to placebo treatment. Each subject was given capsules containing stevioside (250 mg) or placebo thrice daily and followed-up at monthly intervals for 1 year. RESULTS: After 3 months, the systolic and diastolic blood pressure of the stevioside group decreased significantly (systolic: 166.0+/-9.4-152.6+/-6.8 mmHg; diastolic: 104.7 +/-5.2-90.3+/-3.6 mmHg, P<0.05), and the effect persisted during the whole year. Blood biochemistry parameters including lipid and glucose showed no significant changes. No significant adverse effect was observed and quality of life assessment showed no deterioration.

CONCLUSIONS: This study shows that oral stevioside is a well tolerated and effective modality that may be considered as an alternative or supplementary therapy for patients with hypertension.

ଓଃଓଃ

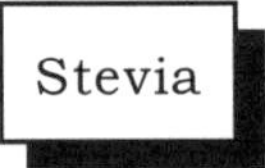

In the journal *Planta Medica* 2001; 67(9):796-9

CN Lee, et al., studied...

"Inhibitory effect of stevioside on calcium influx to produce antihypertension."

Stevioside is a sweet-tasting glycoside occurring abundantly in the leaves of Stevia rebaudiana (Compositae). It has been used popularly in Japan and Brazil as a sugar substitute for decades. Previous study has shown that it lowered blood pressure in spontaneously hypertensive rats (SHRs) when administered intravenously. This study shows that intraperitoneal injection of stevioside 25 mg/kg also has antihypertensive effect in SHRs. In isolated aortic rings from normal rats, stevioside could dose-dependently relax the vasopressin-induced vasoconstriction in both the presence and absence of endothelium. However, stevioside had no effect on phenylephrine- and KCl-induced phasic vasoconstriction. In addition, stevioside lost its influence on vasopressin-induced vasoconstriction in Ca(2+)-free medium. The results indicate that stevioside caused vasorelaxation via an inhibition of Ca(2+) influx into the blood vessel. This phenomenon was further confirmed in cultured aortic smooth muscle cells (A7r5). Using 10(-5) M methylene blue for 15 min, stevioside could still relax 10(-8) M vasopressin-induced vasoconstriction in isolated rat aortic rings, showing that this vasorelaxation effect was not related to nitric oxide. **The present data show that the vasorelexation effect of stevioside was mediated mainly through Ca(2+) influx inhibition.**

ME COMMENTS:

Lee's study demonstrates that the mechanism of action of Stevia to lower blood pressure may be a result of it acting as a natural calcium channel blocker. Calcium channel blockers are a major class of pharmaceuticals which lower blood pressure.

ঙ্গ

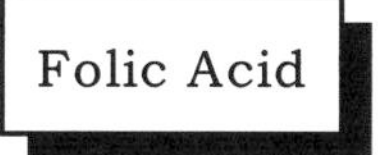

Folic Acid

In the *Journal of the American Medical Association*, 2005;293:320-329.

Dr. John P. Forman, et al., studied...

"Folate Intake and the Risk of Incident Hypertension Among US Women"

Conclusion Higher total folate intake was associated with a decreased risk of incident hypertension, particularly in younger women [and to a lesser extent in older women].

ME COMMENTS:

Dr. John P. Forman, et al. analyzed diet and blood pressure information of more than 150,000 women. None of the women had a history of high blood pressure. Information on the folate intake from dietary sources and supplements was collected from the women and updated every 4 years. The results showed that women aged 27 to 44 years, who ingested at least 1,000 mcg a day of folic acid from their diet and supplements were 46% less likely to develop high blood pressure than women who ingested less than 200 mcg per day. Women aged 43 to 70 years also experienced a blood pressure benefit from folic acid. Among these women, those who had a greater folic acid intake had an 18% lower incidence of high blood pressure. I believe that these findings will also apply to men.

ଔଓଔଓ

Folic Acid

In the journal *BBA - Biochimica et Biophysica Acta* 2005 Nov 15;1726(2):152-9.

P. Stiefel, et al., studied...

"Effects of short-term supplementation with folic acid on different oxidative stress parameters in patients with hypertension."

and found that...

Oxidative stress seems to play an important role in the pathophysiology of essential hypertension. Due to its antioxidant features, we studied the protective action of folic acid in hypertensive patients, their food supplemented for 2 weeks with this vitamin. Several oxidative stress parameters were measured in the serum of these patients....

...The results show that folic acid supplementation improves levels of oxidative stress markers in individuals with hypertension, overall in those patients whose initial parameter values were highest.

ཌྷཌྷ

CoQ10 and Omega3

In the *Journal of Clinical Hypertension* (Greenwich) - 01-MAY-2004; 6(5): 242-8

AJ Wilburn, et al. studied...

"The natural treatment of hypertension"

And found...

The goal of this review is to evaluate the efficacy of commonly available dietary supplements in the treatment of hypertension, using the average blood pressure reduction achieved with the implementation of lifestyle modifications as a standard. For this reason, the authors focus on the antihypertensive potential of these agents rather than pharmacology, pharmacokinetics, adverse effects, or supplement-drug interactions. For the purpose of this review, dietary supplements are defined as exhibiting some evidence of benefit if a systolic blood pressure reduction of 9.0 mm Hg or greater and/or a diastolic blood pressure reduction of 5.0 mm Hg or greater has been observed in previously published, peer-reviewed trials. These defining limits are based on the average blood pressure reduction associated with the implementation of certain lifestyle modifications. **Agents with some evidence of benefit include coenzyme Q10, fish oil, garlic, vitamin C, and L-arginine**.

ME COMMENTS:

Now if only scientists would look at folic acid, bonito peptides, lactobacillus helveticus and stevia, they would get an expanded concept of the effects of natural pharmaceuticals on hypertension.

ଔଔଔଔ

Notes

CHOLESTEROL

Elevated cholesterol levels are a serious medical issue. The American Heart Association (AHA) states that nearly 107 million Americans have total cholesterol of 200 mg/dL or higher, a level at which cardiovascular risk begins to rise. Scientific studies have shown that using statin pharmaceuticals (i.e., Lipitor®, Crestor®, Mevacor®), can lower cholesterol levels. However, these statin pharmaceuticals can cause side effects which impact quality of life including abdominal pain, allergic reactions, back pain, changes in eyesight, constipation, diarrhea, dry eyes, dry skin, hair loss, headache, heartburn, leg cramps, muscle aching or weakness, neuromuscular degeneration, transient memory loss (read about this at www.spacedoc.net) and in rare situations rhabdomyolysis, a muscle condition that can cause kidney failure. These side effects frequently compromise patient willingness to follow the prescribed treatment.

CoQ10 is a **vital** ("indispensable to the continuance of life") substance that assists in the oxidation of nutrients within cells to create energy. It is also highly efficient at protecting internal and external cell membranes against oxidation. **All statin pharmaceuticals interfere with the production of CoQ10 and for this reason, supplementation with CoQ10 is required.**

Red Yeast Rice, Guggullipids, Polycosanols, Omega 3, Phytosterols and Probiotics are just some of the natural pharmaceuticals with scientific evidence of their effectiveness in lowering levels of cholesterol.

Red yeast rice has been used in China for centuries as both a food and as a medicinal substance. Red yeast rice is the fermented product of rice on which red yeast (Monascus Purpureus) has been grown. In Chinese medicine, Red yeast rice is used to promote blood circulation, soothe upset stomach, and invigorate the function of the spleen, the body organ that destroys old blood cells and filters foreign substances. In addition, this dietary supplement has been used traditionally for bruised muscles, hangovers, indigestion, and infant colic.

Cholesterol

The use of Red yeast rice in China was first documented during the Tang Dynasty in 800 AD. It has been used to make rice wine, as a food preservative for maintaining the color and taste of fish and meat, and for its medicinal properties.

The action of the statin pharmaceuticals comes from their ability to inhibit HMG-CoA reductase (hydroxymethylglutaryl-CoA reductase - an enzyme in the pathway for the synthesis of cholesterol and CoQ10). Red yeast rice forms naturally occurring HMG-CoA reductase inhibitors known as monacolins. The medicinal properties of Red yeast rice favorably impact lipid profiles of hypercholesterolemic patients.

Monacolin-K, also known as mevinolin or lovastatin, is the ingredient in Red yeast rice that Merck & Co., pharmaceutical manufacturer of Mevacor® (lovastatin - generic name), asserts is a patented pharmaceutical. However, Red yeast rice contains a family of nine different monacolins, all of which have the ability to inhibit HMG-CoA reductase. Other active ingredients in Red yeast rice, which may be responsible for lowering cholesterol levels include sterols (betasitosterol, campesterol, stigmasterol, sapogenin), isoflavones, and monounsaturated fatty acids.

Dr. Akira Endo, a Japanese biochemist (see about Dr. Endo in "The Wall Street Journal", January 9, 2006 front page), was the first to document the biomolecular action of Red yeast rice, "Monacolin-K, a new hypocholesterolemic agent produced by a Monascus species," *Journal Antibiotics* (Tokyo) 1979;32:852–4. He discovered a strain of Monascus yeast naturally produced a substance that inhibited cholesterol synthesis. He named this strain Monacolin-K (also known as mevinolin and lovastatin).

One of the cholesterol lowering actions of Red yeast rice is a consequence of an inhibitory effect on cholesterol biosynthesis in hepatic cells. It is unclear whether the lipid-lowering effect of Red yeast rice is due solely to the Monacolin-K content, or if the other eight monacolins, sterols, and isoflavones in the Red yeast rice contribute to its cholesterol-lowering effect. One could possibly attribute the success of Red yeast rice in lowering cholesterol levels to a synergistic effect among all of its ingredients.

Many of these natural pharmaceuticals have a synergistic effect ("used esp. of drugs or muscles that work together so the total effect is greater than the sum of the two [or more]").

Red yeast rice is a statin, albeit a natural statin. Therefore, it is subject to all of the potential effects of the statins, i.e. cholesterol lowering and to all of the side effects of the statins. Studies have shown that the side effects of the statins are dose related:

Low dose of statin ≤ than 5 mg = low side effects

High dose of statin ≥ than 40 mg. = potential serious side effects.

Since Red yeast rice has the properties of a statin, it can also potentially inhibit the production of CoQ10; therefore, you must take CoQ10 if you are taking Red yeast rice. A good rule of thumb is that for every 1 mg. of statin, in whatever form, natural or patented pharmaceutical, you should be taking at least 10 mg. of CoQ10.

Red yeast rice is typically available in 400-600 mg. capsules. The Monacolin-K content of most Red yeast rice is less than 0.2%. Therefore, a 0.2% content in a 600 mg. capsule has about 1.2 mg. of Monacolin-K. **I recommend you take no more than 600 mg. of Red yeast rice per day with a Monacolin-K content of no more than 0.2%.** However, if you are taking Red yeast rice as a natural pharmaceutical you must know what the percentage of Monacolin-K is. A higher than 0.2% content will yield more than 1.2 mg per capsule. Compare this 1.2 mg. with doses of pharmaceutical statins which are typically 10-40 mg. per day. We know that statin side effects are dose related and rarely occur in doses of less than 5 mg. per day. The serious side effects do not seem to appear until you exceed doses of 40 mg. per day. It seems that even if Red yeast rice causes the same side effects as the pharmaceutical statins, you would have to take more than 30 (600mg.) capsules per day to experience these side effects.

Phytosterols and Phytostanols represent a group of compounds that are an essential constituent of cell membranes in animals and plants. Cholesterol is actually a sterol of human cells, whereas phytosterols are produced by plants (also called phytosterols and phytostanols). The most common plant sterols are sitosterol, campesterol, and stigmasterol. Plant sterols, although structurally similar to cholesterol, are not synthesized by the human body and are very poorly absorbed. The specific plant sterols that are currently incorporated into foods and supplements are extracted from soybean oil. These plant sterols are esterified to unsaturated fatty acids creating sterol esters which increase lipid solubility, allowing maximal incorporation into a limited amount of fat. Some currently available plant sterols are saturated. They form the stanol derivatives, which are also effective at lowering cholesterol.

Policosanol is the generic term used for a mixture of long chain fatty alcohols, derived chiefly from the waxy coating of sugar cane and used as a dietary supplement to lower cholesterol levels. They belong to a family of wax-like phytochemicals prevalent throughout nature. This substance, used in the dietary supplement industry, is derived from several foods including: sugar cane, rice bran, beeswax, broccoli, spinach, alfalfa and oats.

The main policosanol form in sugar cane is Octacosanol, a long-chain fatty alcohol found in the waxy film that covers the leaves and fruit of the plants that contain it. Sugar cane derived policosanol is a new face on the cholesterol scene in the United States, but is a popular hypocholesterolemic in other countries.

Guggulipids, are derived from a mixture of plant chemicals (ketonic steroids) from the gum resin of Commiphora mukul, called guggulipid, and are an approved treatment for hyperlipidemia in India. They have been a mainstay in traditional Indian herbal medicine (Ayurveda) therapy for preventing high cholesterol and atherosclerosis. Clinical studies indicate them to be effective in the treatment of elevated cholesterol, elevated triglyceride levels and elevated LDL (bad cholesterol) levels. Studies have also shown that LDL oxidation, which is the main cause of plaque build up in the arteries, can be prevented or at least decreased by the antioxidant activity of guggul. Clinical studies on guggul indicate that its hypolipidemic activity (decreasing cholesterol and other lipids) can be attributed to more than one mechanism. Three of the possible mechanisms include inhibition of cholesterol biosynthesis, enhancing the rate of excretion of cholesterol and promoting rapid degradation of cholesterol.

Guggul is typically manufactured in a standardized form that provides a fixed amount of guggulipid, the presumed active ingredient in guggul. Guggul helps reduce high cholesterol, because it lowers harmful LDL (low-density lipoproteins) while elevating the beneficial HDL (high-density lipoproteins). It helps prevent blood platelet aggregation and breaks up blood clots. Thus guggul can be used, not only to lower bad cholesterol, but can also be used as a preventative against heart disease and stroke.

It is important to monitor your cholesterol levels to make sure that the natural pharmaceuticals that you are using are exerting the proper cholesterol lowering effects.

Even though natural pharmaceuticals are available over the counter and do not require a written prescription, it is highly recommended that you use them under the supervision of a licensed medical professional.

The following scientific studies document the evidence based approach to using various natural pharmaceuticals that may lower your cholesterol levels.

ଔଓଔଓ

Cholesterol Levels as a Predictor of Future Heart Attacks

In the Journal of the American Medical Association, *JAMA*. 2005;294:326-333.

Dr. Paul M Ridker, et al. studied...

"Non–HDL Cholesterol, Apolipoproteins A-I and B100, Standard Lipid Measures, Lipid Ratios, and CRP as Risk Factors for Cardiovascular Disease in Women"

and found that...

"Non–HDL-C and the ratio of total cholesterol to HDL-C were as good as or better than apolipoprotein fractions in the prediction of future cardiovascular events."

ME Comments:

Dr. Ridker found that no test was better at predicting future heart disease related complications such as heart attack and stroke than cholesterol levels in women. I suspect that these findings will also apply to men.

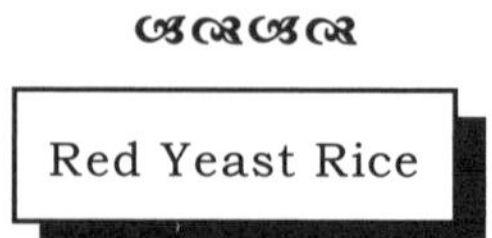

In the *American Journal of Clinical Nutrition*, Vol. 69, No. 2, 231-236, February 1999

David Heber, et al., studied...

"Cholesterol-lowering effects of a proprietary Chinese red-yeast-rice dietary supplement"

Background: We examined the cholesterol-lowering effects of a proprietary Chinese red-yeast-rice supplement in an American population consuming a diet similar to the American Heart Association Step I diet using a double-blind, placebo-controlled, prospectively randomized 12-wk controlled trial at a university research center.

Results: Total cholesterol concentrations decreased significantly between baseline and 8 wk in the red-yeast-rice--treated group compared with the placebo-treated group [(x ± SD) 6.57 ± 0.93 mmol/L (254 ± 36 mg/dL) to 5.38 ± 0.80 mmol/L (208 ± 31 mg/dL); P < 0.001]. LDL cholesterol and total triacylglycerol were also reduced with the supplement. HDL cholesterol did not change significantly.

Conclusions: Red yeast rice significantly reduces total cholesterol, LDL cholesterol, and total triacylglycerol concentrations compared with placebo and provides a new, novel, food-based approach to lowering cholesterol in the general population.

Excerpts from the Discussion:

In 1979, Endo A. (Monacolin-K, "a new hypocholesterolemic agent produced by a Monascus species." *J Antibiot* (Tokyo) 1979;32:852–4) discovered that a strain of Monascus yeast naturally produced a substance that inhibits cholesterol synthesis, which he named Monacolin-K (also known as mevinolin and lovastatin), as well as a family of 8 monacolin-related substances with the ability to inhibit 3-hydroxy-3-methylglutaryl coenzyme A (HMG-CoA) reductase. In addition to the inhibitors of HMG-CoA reductase, Red yeast rice has been found to contain sterols (ß-sitosterol, campesterol, stigmasterol, and sapogenin), isoflavones and isoflavone glycosides, and monounsaturated fatty acids. The quantities of the family of inhibitors of HMG-CoA reductase contained in Red yeast rice are inadequate to explain the magnitude of the lowering of cholesterol observed in this study by comparison with evaluations of lovastatin. The Monacolin-K content is only 0.2%, or {approx}5 mg. Therefore, 5 mg is the relevant comparison to 20–40 mg lovastatin. At this concentration, the mixture of monacolins and other substances present in the Red yeast rice may have some effect on cholesterol biosynthesis not explained by the Monacolin-K content. The effect is unlikely to be due solely to a single species of monacolin, but rather to result from a combination of actions of monacolins and other substances in the Red yeast rice...

...The benefits of statin drugs on the primary prevention of heart disease and in the secondary prevention of recurrent heart disease have been shown in several large, prospective clinical trials. These studies have increased interest in the use of statins for heart disease prevention, such as for individuals with hypercholesterolemia and modest cholesterol elevations. Although it is acknowledged that side effects with statins are rare and **dose related**, there are data indicating that some statins may cause liver function abnormalities and, under certain circumstances, rhabdomyolysis....

...This study was an important first step in establishing that the observed effects of Red yeast rice in China were not due to diet alone but could be clearly related to this Chinese red-yeast-rice dietary supplement in a placebo-controlled, randomized trial. This study also established the need for a study on the long-term safety and efficacy of this supplement in a larger population. The effects observed on triacylglycerol concentrations and HDL-cholesterol concentrations in the Chinese studies also need to be examined in future studies by using carefully controlled diets in appropriately selected populations.

ME COMMENTS:

In this trial Dr. Heber used 2400 mg. per day of Red yeast rice. The Monacolin-K percentage in his study was 0.2%. Therefore, the equivalent amount of statin would be 4.8 mg. This is in contrast to the 10-40 mg. of pharmaceutical statin that most physicians prescribe for elevated cholesterol levels which represents 2-10 times the amount to achieve the same results as Dr. Heber. Dr. Heber notes that "The effect [lowering cholesterol levels] is unlikely to be due solely to a single species of monacolin, but rather to result from a combination of actions of monacolins and other substances in the Red yeast rice..." In addition to Monacolin-K, Red yeast rice has eight other monacolins, along with phytosterols which may also be responsible for its cholesterol lowering properties.

It makes sense to add all of the other cholesterol reducing agents together, therefore, I recommend no more than 600 mg. of Red yeast rice per day, yielding 1.2 mg of natural statin, together with CoQ10, guggulipids, policosanol, phytosterols and phytostanols.

I don't think the point can be emphasized enough that statins, natural or pharmaceutical, have potential side effects which are dose related. Therefore, I recommend the lowest dose of Red yeast rice known to have beneficial effect, 600 mg per day, yielding 1.2 mg. of natural statin.

See Appendix C for excerpts from Dr. David Heber's testimony before the House Government Reform Committee.

ଔଓଔଓ

Red Yeast Rice

In the *European Journal of Endocrinology*, Vol 153, Issue 5, 679-686.

Lin Cheng-Chieh, et al., studied...

"Efficacy and safety of Monascus purpureus Went rice in subjects with hyperlipidemia"

Objective: The purpose of this study was to assess the lipid-lowering effect of Monascus purpureus Went rice on serum lipids in patients with hyperlipidemia, and to assess its safety by reporting adverse events and clinical laboratory measurements.

Design and methods: This was a randomized, double-blind, placebo-controlled study. In all, 79 patients (aged 23–65 years) with a mean baseline low-density lipoprotein cholesterol (LDL-C) level of 5.28 mmol/l (203.9 mg/dl) received a twice daily dose of placebo or Monascus purpureus Went rice (600 mg) for 8 weeks.

Conclusion: Monascus purpureus Went rice significantly reduced LDL-C, total cholesterol, triglycerides and apolipoprotein B levels, and was well tolerated in patients with hyperlipidemia. However, this study only provides data from an 8-week trial and long-term safety and efficacy data are needed.

ଔଓଔଓ

Red Yeast Rice

In the *American Heart Journal* 147•3•2004

Kelly L. Miller, et al., studied...

"Complementary and alternative medicine in cardiovascular disease: a review of biologically based approaches"

Excerpt

...Red yeast rice has been a food staple and folk remedy in the Far East for thousands of years. It was noted in the 1970s that a product of the yeast, Monacolin-K (lovastatin), inhibited HMG-CoA reductase. The concentration of lovastatin in Red yeast rice varies, but averages 0.4% by weight.

In the preliminary report of a multicenter study of 187 subjects presented by Rippe et al at the 39th Annual Conference on Cardiovascular Disease Epidemiology and Prevention in Orlando, Fla, in 1999, **Red yeast rice lowered total cholesterol levels 16.4%, LDL cholesterol levels 21.0%, triglyceride levels 24.5%, and the total cholesterol to HDL cholesterol ratio 17.7% and increased HDL cholesterol levels 14.6%.**

ଔଓଔଓ

Red Yeast Rice and CoQ10

In the *British Journal of Nutrition* 2005 Jan;93(1):131-5.

HT Yang, et al., studied...

"Acute administration of red yeast rice (Monascus purpureus) depletes tissue coenzyme Q(10) levels in ICR mice."

In this study, we attempted to evaluate the effect of administration of a high quantity of Red yeast rice on coenzyme Q10 (CoQ10) synthesis in the tissues of ICR mice. Eighty-eight adult male ICR mice were housed and divided into control and experimental groups for Red yeast rice treatment. Animals were gavaged with a low (1 g/kg body weight) or a high dose (5 g/kg body weight, approximately five times the typical recommended human dose) of Red yeast rice dissolved in soyabean oil. After gavagement, animals of the control group were immediately killed; mice of the experimental groups (eight for each subgroup) were killed at different time intervals of 0.5, 1, 1.5, 4 and 24 h. The liver, heart and kidney were taken for analysis of Monacolin-K (liver only) and CoQ10 analysis. Liver and heart CoQ10 levels declined dramatically in both groups administered Red yeast rice, especially in the high-dose group, within 30 min. After 24 h, the levels of hepatic and cardiac CoQ10 were still reduced. A similar trend was also observed in the heart, but the inhibitory effect began after 90 min. The higher dose of Red yeast rice presented a greater suppressive effect than did the lower dose on tissue CoQ10 levels.

In conclusion, acute Red yeast rice gavage suppressed hepatic and cardiac CoQ10 levels in rodents; furthermore, the inhibitory effect was responsive to the doses administered.

Excerpts from Discussion:

...In our study, we applied five times the human recommended dosages (Red yeast rice) in ICR mice. No histological damage, or even skin irritation was observed in any animal. According to such a description, it is believed that, with low citrinin content, no safety concerns exist for the recommended dosages of Red yeast rice....

ME COMMENTS:

Red yeast rice will lower CoQ10 levels. This response is dose related; therefore, if you are taking Red yeast rice as a natural pharmaceutical you must add CoQ10. For every mg. of statin that you are taking, you need at least 10 mg. of CoQ10. Remember, most 600 mg capsules of Red yeast rice contain 0.2% natural statins - i.e. 1.2 mg of statin per capsule. That will require supplementation with at least 12 mg. of Co-Q10.

☙❧☙❧

CoQ10 and Statins

In the journal *Archives of Neurology*. 2004;61:889-892.

Dr. Tatjana Rundek, et al, studied...

"Atorvastatin Decreases the Coenzyme Q10 Level in the Blood of Patients at Risk for Cardiovascular Disease and Stroke"

Background: Statins [Lipitor®, Crestor®, Mevacor®, etc.].... are widely used for the treatment of hypercholesterolemia and coronary heart disease and for the prevention of stroke. There have been various adverse effects, most commonly affecting muscle and ranging from myalgia to rhabdomyolysis. These adverse effects may be due to a coenzyme Q10 (CoQ10) deficiency because inhibition of cholesterol biosynthesis also inhibits the synthesis of CoQ10.

Objective: To measure CoQ10 levels in blood from hypercholesterolemic subjects before and after exposure to atorvastatin calcium, 80 mg/d, for 14 and 30 days.

Conclusions: Even brief exposure to atorvastatin [Lipitor®] causes a marked decrease in blood CoQ10 concentration. Widespread inhibition of CoQ10 synthesis could explain the most commonly reported adverse effects of statins, especially exercise intolerance, myalgia, and myoglobinuria.

ME COMMENTS:

CoQ10 is a vital substance. All of the statin family of drugs use one of the same metabolic pathways as CoQ10 and thereby block some of the CoQ10 production. If you are taking any type of statin drug, you must take a CoQ10 supplement. Even though Red yeast rice is a natural statin, and there is no scientific evidence that Red yeast rice interferes with the production of CoQ10 I recommend that if you are taking Red yeast rice you should supplement it with CoQ10.

CoQ10 and Statins

In the journal *Archives of Neurology*. 2005;62:1709-1712.

Dr. Costanza Lamperti, et al., studied...

"Muscle Coenzyme Q10 Level in Statin-Related Myopathy"

Background: Statin drugs (3-hydroxy-3-methylglutaryl coenzyme A reductase inhibitors) reduce the level of cholesterol by inhibiting the synthesis of mevalonate, an intermediary in the cholesterol biosynthetic pathway. Use of statin drugs has been associated with a variety of skeletal muscle–related complaints. Coenzyme Q10 (CoQ10), a component of the mitochondrial respiratory chain, is also synthesized from mevalonate, and decreased muscle CoQ10 concentration may have a role in the pathogenesis of statin drug–related myopathy....

...Conclusion: These data suggest that statin drug–related myopathy is associated with a mild decrease in muscle CoQ10 concentration, which does not cause histochemical or biochemical evidence of mitochondrial myopathy or morphologic evidence of apoptosis in most patients.

❧❧❧❧

Phytosterols and Phytostanols

In the journal *New England Journal of Medicine*. Volume 333:1308-1312

Dr. Tatu A. Miettinen, et al. studied...

"Reduction of Serum Cholesterol with Sitostanol-Ester Margarine in a Mildly Hypercholesterolemic Population"

Background: Dietary plant sterols, especially sitostanol, reduce serum cholesterol by inhibiting cholesterol absorption. Soluble sitostanol may be more effective than a less soluble preparation. We tested the tolerability and cholesterol-lowering effect of margarine containing sitostanol ester in a population with mild hypercholesterolemia.

Methods: We conducted a one-year, randomized, double-blind study in 153 randomly selected subjects with mild hypercholesterolemia. Fifty-one consumed margarine without sitostanol ester (the control group), and 102 consumed margarine containing sitostanol ester (1.8 or 2.6 g of sitostanol per day).

and found that...

Conclusions: Substituting sitostanol-ester margarine for part of the daily fat intake in subjects with mild hypercholesterolemia was effective in lowering serum total cholesterol and LDL cholesterol.

ME COMMENTS:

More scientific evidence that natural products like phytosterols lower cholesterol levels.

ഗ്ദ ഗ്ദ

Phytosterols and Phytostanols

Food and Drug Administration September 5, 2000

"FDA AUTHORIZES NEW CORONARY HEART DISEASE HEALTH CLAIM FOR PLANT STEROL AND PLANT STANOL ESTERS"

The FDA has authorized use of labeling health claims about the role of plant sterol or plant stanol esters in reducing the risk of coronary heart disease (CHD) for foods containing these substances. This interim final rule is based on FDA's conclusion that plant sterol esters and plant stanol esters may reduce the risk of CHD by lowering blood cholesterol levels.

...This new health claim is based on evidence that plant sterol or plant stanol esters may help to reduce the risk of CHD. Plant sterols are present in small quantities in many fruits, vegetables, nuts, seeds, cereals, legumes, and other plant sources. Plant stanols occur naturally in even smaller quantities from some of the same sources. For example, both plant sterols and stanols are found in vegetable oils.

ME COMMENTS:

Evidence from the FDA that phytosterols and phytostanols lower cholesterol levels. It is no longer just the alternative medicine doctors who are recommending natural alternatives for lowering cholesterol levels.

ଓଡଓଡ

Phytosterols and Phytostanols

In the journal *Pharmacotherapy*. 2005; 25 (2): 171-183.

Judy T. Chen, et al., studied...

"Meta Analysis of Natural Therapies for Hyperlipidemia: Plant Sterols and Stanols vs. Policosanol."

Study Objective: To compare the efficacy and safety of plant sterols and stanols as well as policosanol in the treatment of coronary heart disease, as measured by a reduction in low-density lipoprotein cholesterol (LDL) levels.

Conclusion: Plant sterols and stanols and policosanol are well tolerated and safe; however, policosanol is more effective than plant sterols and stanols for LDL level reduction and more favorably alters the lipid profile, approaching antilipemic drug efficacy.

ME COMMENTS:

This study shows that policosanol is more effective in lowering cholesterol levels than sterols and stanols. Why not put them all together to achieve a synergistic effect?

ଓଡଓଡ

Policosanol

In the *American Heart Journal.* 2002 Feb;143(2):356-65.

I Gouni-Berthold, et al., studied...

"Policosanol: clinical pharmacology and therapeutic significance of a new lipid-lowering agent."

Policosanol is a mixture of higher primary aliphatic alcohols isolated from sugar cane wax, whose main component is octacosanol. The mixture has been shown to lower cholesterol in animal models, healthy volunteers, and patients with type II hypercholesterolemia....

RESULTS: At doses of 10 to 20 mg per day, policosanol lowers total cholesterol by 17% to 21% and low-density lipoprotein (LDL) cholesterol by 21% to 29% and raises high-density lipoprotein cholesterol by 8% to 15%. Because higher doses have not been tested up to now, it cannot be excluded that effectiveness may be even greater. Daily doses of 10 mg of policosanol have been shown to be equally effective in lowering total or LDL cholesterol as the same dose of simvastatin or pravastatin. Triglyceride levels are not influenced by policosanol. At dosages of up to 20 mg per day, policosanol is safe and well tolerated, as studies of >3 years of therapy indicate. There is evidence from in vitro studies that policosanol may inhibit hepatic cholesterol synthesis at a step before mevalonate generation, but direct inhibition of the hydroxy-methylglutaryl-coenzyme A reductase is unlikely. Animal studies suggest that LDL catabolism may be enhanced, possibly through receptor-mediated mechanisms, but the precise mechanism of action is not understood yet. Policosanol has additional beneficial properties such as effects on smooth muscle cell proliferation, platelet aggregation, and LDL peroxidation. Data on efficacy determined by clinical end points such as rates of cardiac events or cardiac mortality are lacking.

CONCLUSIONS: Policosanol seems to be a very promising phytochemical alternative to classic lipid-lowering agents such as the statins and deserves further evaluation.

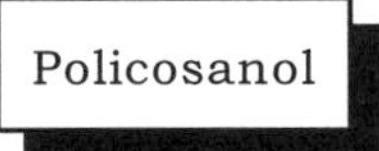

From *Clinical Drug Investigation™* 25(11):701-707, 2005.

Željko Reiner, et. al., studied...

"Effects of Rice Policosanol on Serum Lipoproteins, Homocysteine, Fibrinogen and C-Reactive Protein in Hypercholesterolaemic Patients"

and found that...

Results: Rice policosanol significantly reduced plasma total cholesterol from 7.37 ± 1.42 mmol/L to 6.99 ± 1.33 mmol/L (p = 0.007) and increased Apo AI from 1.49 ± 0.39 mmol/L to 1.58 ± 0.38 mmol/L (p = 0.037) but did not change plasma triglycerides, HDL, HDL2, HDL3 and LDL cholesterol, ox-LDL, Lp(a), Apo B, fibrinogen, homocysteine or CRP levels.

Conclusion: Rice policosanol 10 mg/day moderately decreased plasma total cholesterol and increased Apo AI. Rice policosanol was also well tolerated, with no drug-related effects on safety parameters such as serum aminotransferases and creatine phosphokinase detected or found on physical examination.

ꟹꟹ

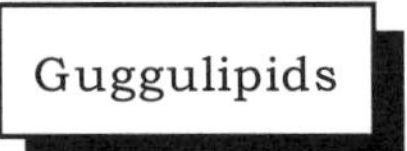

In the journal *Science*, 2002; 296(5573):1703-6

NL Urizar, et al., studied...

"A natural product that lowers cholesterol as an antagonist ligand for FXR."

Extracts of the resin of the guggul tree (Commiphora mukul) lower LDL (low-density lipoprotein) cholesterol levels in humans. The plant sterol guggulsterone [4,17(20)-pregna-diene-3,16-dione] is the active agent in this extract. We show that guggulsterone is a highly efficacious antagonist of the farnesoid X receptor (FXR), a nuclear hormone receptor that is activated by bile acids. Guggulsterone treatment decreases hepatic cholesterol in wild-type mice fed a high-cholesterol diet but is not effective in FXR-null mice. Thus, we propose that inhibition of FXR activation is the basis for the cholesterol-lowering activity of guggulsterone. Other natural products with specific biologic effects may modulate the activity of FXR or other relatively promiscuous nuclear hormone receptors.

ꕥꕥꕥꕥ

Boswellia

In the *Indian Journal of Experimental Biology*, 2005; 43(6):509-16

RS Pandey, et al., studied...

"Extract of gum resins of Boswellia serrata L. inhibits lipopolysaccharide induced nitric oxide production in rat macrophages along with hypolipidemic property."

Boswellia serrata, Linn F (Burseraceae) is commonly used in Indian system of medicine (Ayurvedic) as an anti-inflammatory, analgesic, anti-arthritic and anti-proliferative agent. This study was planned to investigate the water-soluble fraction of the oleoresin gum of Boswellia serrata (BS extract) on lipopolysaccharide (LPS) induced nitric oxide (NO) production by macrophages under in vivo and in vitro conditions. In the previous condition, rats were fed on atherogenic diet (2.5% cholesterol, 1% cholic acid, 15.7 % saturated fat) along with the BS extract for 90 days. Blood was collected for lipid profile and toxicological safety parameters. Peritoneal macrophages were isolated and cultured to see the LPS induced NO production. Under in vivo experiment, BS extract significantly reduced serum total cholesterol (38-48 %), increased serum high-density lipoprotein- cholesterol (HDL-cholesterol, 22-30%). Under in vitro experiments with thioglycolate activated macrophages, it inhibited LPS induced (NO) production with IC 50 value at 662 ng /ml. Further, this fraction, in the dose of 15 mg/ 100 g body wt for 90 days, did not show any increase in serum glutamate-pyruvate transaminase (SGPT) and blood urea, in normal control animals. However, it significantly reversed the raised SGPT and blood urea in the atherogenic diet-fed animals. Transverse section of liver and kidney also supported its protective effect. **Thus it may be concluded that water extract of Boswellia serrata possesses strong hypocholesterolemic property along with increase in serum HDL.** It inhibits the LPS induced NO production by the activated rat peritoneal macrophages and show hepato-protective and reno-protective property.

ME COMMENTS:

Boswellia also has anti-inflammatory properties and is useful for muscle and joint pain (see chapter on muscle and joint pain).

ଓଷଓଷ

Policosanol and Omega3

In the journal *Drugs in R&D.* 2005; 6(4):207-19

G Castaño, et al., studied...

"Effects of addition of policosanol to omega-3 fatty acid therapy on the lipid profile of patients with type II hypercholesterolaemia."

CONCLUSIONS: Policosanol 5 or 10 mg/day administered concomitantly with omega-3 FA 1 g/day improved LDL-C, TC and HDL-C, maintained the reduction in TG attributable to omega-3 FA monotherapy, and was well tolerated. Treatment with omega-3 FA + policosanol could be useful for regulating lipid profile in patients with type II hypercholesterolaemia, but further studies involving larger sample sizes are needed before definitive conclusions can be drawn.

ଓଷଓଷ

Policosanol & Red Yeast Rice

In the journal *Arzneimittel-Forschung.* 2005; 55(6):312-7

I. Setnikar, et al., studied...

"Antiatherosclerotic efficacy of policosanol, red yeast rice extract and astaxanthin [an antioxidant also called Vitamin X] in the rabbit."

The effects of policosanol (P), of extract of Red yeast rice (rice fermented with Monascus purpureus) (RYE) and of astaxanthin (A) (constituents of Armolipid) were investigated in a model of experimental atherosclerosis provoked in the rabbit by atherogenic cholesterol-enriched feed (ACEF). P and RYE and their combination were able to lower the increase of serum total cholesterol and of LDL cholesterol elicited by 3-month feeding with ACEF. They also were able to reduce the increase of blood malondialdehyde (MDA), a tracer of lipid peroxidation by the free radicals released by ACEF. **When combined, the substances developed either additive or potentiated effects, supporting the rationale of their combination.** Remarkable was the protective effect on lipid infiltration in the aortic wall provoked by ACEF, which was reduced by P and by RYE and almost completely prevented by the addition of A to the P-RYE combination.

The results support the rationale of a combination of P, RYE and A as a useful food supplement in hyperlipemic patients.

ME COMMENTS:

Since there have been no scientific studies showing antioxidants as lowering cholesterol levels, the cholesterol lowering shown in this study was probably due to the policosanol and Red yeast rice. Many of these natural pharmaceuticals have a synergistic effect ("used esp. of drugs or muscles that work together so the total effect is greater than the sum of the two [or more]")

ꟹ

Cholesterol
Probiotics and Prebiotics

In the journal *Applied and Environmental Microbiology* 01-APR-2005; 71(4): 1745-53

MT Liong, et al., studied...

"Optimization of cholesterol removal by probiotics in the presence of prebiotics by using a response surface method."

Abstract:

Lactobacillus casei ASCC 292 was grown in the presence of six prebiotics, namely, sorbitol, mannitol, maltodextrin, high-amylose maize, fructooligosaccharide (FOS), and inulin, in order to determine the combination of probiotic and prebiotics that would remove the highest level of cholesterol. **A first-order model showed that the combination of L. casei ASCC 292, FOS, and maltodextrin was the most efficient for the removal of cholesterol...**

ME COMMENTS:

MT Liong's study shows that a combination of probiotics with prebiotics was the most effective means for lowering cholesterol levels. This is the reason why I recommend probiotics with FOS as a treatment for high cholesterol levels.

☙❧☙❧

Notes

PROBIOTIC BACTERIA
Friendly Bacteria

The important thing in science is not so much to obtain new facts as to discover new ways of thinking about them."

Sir William Bragg (1862-1942)**

Probiotic means "for life" (as opposed to antibiotic which means "anti life").

Probiotics are living microorganisms (bacterial or yeast) which, upon ingestion in certain numbers, exert health benefits beyond inherent basic nutrition.

All known probiotic bacteria belong to the group called lactic acid bacteria, which in this context includes the species Lactococcus, Lactobacillus, Streptococcus, Leuconostoc, Pediococcus, Bifidobacterium and Enterococcus.

To be a successful probiotic, the bacteria must fulfill the following criteria:

- Non-pathogenic
- Resistant to technologic processes and exert minimal sensory influence on the probiotic food
- Survive passage through the gastrointestinal tract (resistant to gastric acidity and bile acids)
- Adhere to the gut epithelial tissue and possess growth capability
- Provide health benefits

***Pioneer British scientist in solid-state physics who was a joint winner (with his son Sir Lawrence Bragg) of the Nobel Prize for Physics in 1915 for his research.*

Probiotic Bacteria

Different strains of probiotic bacteria have been shown to ameliorate certain medical conditions. The current scientific research indicates that multiple strains of probiotic bacteria can be combined into one capsule, with the addition of a prebiotic like FOS or MOS to provide a synergistic effect. Lactobacillus Helvitucus has been shown to lower blood pressure, Lactobacillus Rhammosus, and Bifidobacterium Bifidum have been shown to prevent Rotovirus diarrhea. Lactobacillus Rhammosus and Saccromyces Boullardii have been shown to prevent C-Difficile diarrhea. Lactobacillus Casei, has been shown to lower cholesterol levels. Saccromyces Boullardii, Lactobacillus Acidophilus, Bifidobacterium Bifidum, and Streptoccus Thermophilus have been shown to prevent travelers diarrhea. Lactobacillus Acidophilus, Bifidobacterium Bifidum and Lactobacillus Rhammosus have been shown to prevent other types of diarrhea, as well as to modulate the immune system.

Inside each of us live vast numbers of friendly bacteria without which we could not remain in good health. Before looking at the amazing things they do, reflect on just how many of them we house. There are several trillion friendly bacteria in each person (more than all the cells in the body) divided among more than 400 species, most of them inhabiting the digestive tract. If they were all placed together the total weight of these "friendly" bacteria would come to nearly four pounds. In fact, about a third of the fecal matter (water removed) which you pass consists of dead or viable bacteria.

These bacteria are not parasites. They do not just take up residence and do nothing in return, but perform many important functions in the body. We live in true symbiosis with them. As long as we provide them with a reasonable diet and as long as they remain in good health, these bacteria provide excellent service in return.

Some of the different validated functions of Probiotics are that they create:

- Milk-digesting enzyme lactase which helps digest dairy products
- Nutrients, i.e. Folic Acid, Niacin, Riboflavin, Vitamin B6 & Vitamin B12

- Antibacterial substances which kill or deactivate hostile disease-causing bacteria

They help to:

- Improve the efficiency of the digestive tract
- Reduce high cholesterol levels
- Reduce high blood pressure levels
- Play an important part in the development of a baby's digestive function and immune system. Bifidobacteria infantis is acquired from breast milk. When it is in poor supply allergies and malabsorption problems are more common
- Protect against radiation damage and deactivate many toxic pollutants
- Recycle estrogen (a female hormone) which reduces menopausal symptoms and osteoporosis
- Bifidobacteria and acidophilus have been shown to have powerful anticarcinogenic features which are active against certain tumors

Therapeutically they have been shown to be useful in the treatment of:

- acne
- psoriasis
- eczema
- allergies
- migraine
- gout
- rheumatic and arthritic conditions
- cystitis
- candidiasis
- colitis
- irritable bowel syndrome
- some forms of cancer
- AAD (antibiotic associated diarrhea)
- constipation
- Traveler's Diarrhea

There are two components to the probiotic family: Probiotic Bacteria (friendly bacteria) and Probiotic Yeast (friendly yeast, i.e.

Saccromyces Boullardii). Even though the mechanism of action is different, the outcome is the same, an increase in the amount of healthy bacteria in our system. Thereby, preventing the condition of dysbiosis (an imbalance of bacteria in the GI tract, involving an overgrowth of unhealthy organisms, including candida albicans and a variety of other harmful bacteria and parasites). Dysbiosis is a cofactor, if not a primary cause of: cholitis, digestive problems, fatigue, food allergy, intestinal gas and bloating, irritable bowel syndrome, yeast infections, hypertension and high cholesterol. This is not a complete list, but is enough to give a general idea of the problems associated with dysbiosis.

The other components of the probiotic story are Short Chain Fatty Acids (SCFAs) and Prebiotics. Prebiotics are food for the friendly bacteria (see chapter on prebiotics). SCFAs are one of the most important products of friendly bacteria (see chapter on SCFAs).

Why is there so much interest in probiotics and why has it become such a hot topic in the scientific literature? A literature search produces over 100 articles written in the last six months. If you do a *Google* search for probiotics today, March 2006, you will get 2,170,000 hits. Just six months earlier there were only 600,000 hits.

Why?... Because despite over 50 years of antibiotic use, infectious disease remains a major cause of death. Hospital infection rates are not declining, multi drug resistant bacteria continue to emerge as the antibiotic pipeline dries up and pathogenic micro-organisms are being linked with the worsening of many chronic diseases. The scientific community is playing a major role in the ever growing number of studies providing evidence that probiotics can alleviate some diseases.

There is a long history of health claims concerning living microorganisms in food, particularly lactic acid bacteria (lactobacillus). In a Persian version of the Old Testament Genesis 18:8, "and he (Abraham) took curd and milk," Abraham may have owed his longevity to the consumption of sour milk. In 76 BC the Roman historian, Plinius, recommended the administration of fermented milk products for the treatment of gastroenteritis.

We know that the intestine, besides being a digestive organ, affects the immune system. The over 500 trillion friendly bacteria that live in our intestine communicate with each other, modulating many of the functions of our body. A decrease in the number of these bacteria, either because of antibiotic use (antibiotics will destroy healthy bacteria as well as pathogenic bacteria) or from lack of food containing healthy bacteria (all processed food is sterilized and pasteurized, killing all bacteria including friendly bacteria). The primary use of probiotics is to restore the normal flora in the intestines. They do this first by competing with other organisms for nutrients. They secrete SCFAs decreasing the pH of the vagina and intestines, making the environment less favorable for the pathogenic bacteria to thrive.

In the past, food preservation was accomplished through fermentation, a process that adds a host of beneficial microorganisms to food. However, fermentation is an inconsistent process; therefore, commercial food processors developed techniques like pasteurization (which kills all microorganisms), to help standardize more consistent yields.

Scientific studies have demonstrated that a lack of healthy bacteria can be one of the causes that lead to medical problems such as: food allergies, bacterial vaginosis of pregnancy, irritable bowel syndrome, urinary tract infections, yeast infections, intestinal infections, allergy, asthma, genital infections, elevated blood pressure, (all lactobacilli have ace inhibitor properties, thereby lowering blood pressure), elevated cholesterol levels, recurrent ear and bladder infections, antibiotic associated diarrhea, and protection of the newborn against atopic disease. The scientific literature has documented that many of these problems can be reversed with the use of probiotics.

All combinations of live, friendly bacteria will bring about some of the reported health benefits. As we learn more about friendly bacteria we will see scientists isolate unique strains of friendly bacteria which will be used to treat specific conditions.

I recommend **Probiotics** and **Digestive Enzymes** for patients who have any type of gastrointestinal complaint, hypertension, high cholesterol levels and for health maintenance. I have included just a handful of the hundreds of studies available on probiotics. Dr. Kelly Karpa's book *Bacteria for Breakfast* provides an indepth understanding of the actions of probiotics. Read more, research more and most importantly take your probiotics daily.

The following scientific studies document the evidence based approach to using various probiotic bacteria for many conditions.

ଓଡ଼ଓଡ଼

Probiotics and Pregnancy

In *The Israel Medical Association Journal* 2002;4:357-360

Dr. Eliezer Shalev studied...

"Ingestion of Probiotics: Optional Treatment of Bacterial Vaginosis [BV] in Pregnancy"

And found that...

Bacterial vaginosis is the primary cause of abnormal vaginal discharge in women of reproductive age.

Synopsis

In epidemiologic studies of women with vaginitis, at least 30 to 50% of all women have BV. The predominant bacteria in the normal vaginal flora are Lactobacillus species, which establish a low vaginal pH by producing lactic acid. Some types of Lactobacillus also generate hydrogen peroxide. The low pH value and the presence of hydrogen peroxide inhibit the growth of most other microorganisms. In women with BV, the vaginal flora are altered by replacement of the normal peroxide-producing Lactobacillus species with high concentrations of anaerobic bacteria (e.g., Mobiluncus sp. Bacteroides sp.), Gardnerella vaginalis, and Mycoplasma hominis. Although BV is the most prevalent cause of vaginal discharge or mal-odor; half of the women who meet the clinical diagnostic criteria for BV are asymptomatic.

In conclusion, the possibility of using lactobacilli is promising. Although scientific confirmation is still needed, probiotics may be especially important for reducing the preterm birth rate in pregnant women. It has been claimed that intrauterine infection with BV may antedate the pregnancy. Probiotics can safely be used before pregnancy or in the first trimester. Moreover, it may be used as an adjunctive therapy in the second trimester, avoiding potential side effects and teratogenicity of standard treatments. Probiotics may well be the answer.

ME COMMENTS:

We are beginning to appreciate the risks of antibiotics, as well as their lack of effectiveness due to bacteria becoming resistant.

ଓଷଓଷ

Probiotics and Allergy

In the *Current Opinion in Allergy & Clinical Immunology.* 3(1):15-20, February 2003.

Dr. Marko Kalliomaki, et al.,

"Role of intestinal flora in the development of allergy."

Abstract:

Purpose of review: The frequency of allergic diseases is increasing worldwide. Experimental and clinical studies have linked a reduced number of early infections to this trend. The gastrointestinal system, which comprises the largest lymphoid tissue and microbial reservoir of the body, has received more attention during the last few years as a potential determiner in the development of atopic disease.

Recent findings: Alterations in intestinal microbiota have been detected both in infants suffering from allergic disease and in those later developing the disorder. Delay in the compositional development of Bifidobacterium and Lactobacillus in gut microflora was a general finding in allergic children. In a subsequent study, perinatal administration of lactobacilli halved the later development of atopic eczema during the first 2 years of life. Specific strains of the healthy gut microbiota have been shown to induce the production of IL-10 and transforming growth factor-[beta], which possess an important regulative role in the development of allergic type immune response. Probiotics also strengthen gut defence barrier mechanisms and reduce antigen load in the gut. Pattern recognition receptors in intestinal epithelial and antigen-presenting cells have been demonstrated to mediate a continuing dialogue between host and gut microbiota.

Summary: Despite several promising findings, the exact role of gut normal microbiota in the development of allergy remains to be elucidated. For successful interventions, more data concerning a communication between host and specific microbial species are needed.

ME COMMENTS:

It is becoming clear that the intestinal flora have active roles in the development of allergy. During the first two years of life, low amounts of healthy bacteria seem to lead to increased allergy in children . How do we stop this? Lower Cesarean Section rates, more breast-feeding, and more use of probiotics.

ꕥꕥꕥꕥ

Probiotics and Non-Intestinal Infection

In the *British Journal of Nutrition,* Volume 88, Supplement s1, September 2002, pp. 59-66(8)

Dr. M. de Vrese, et al. Studied

"Probiotics and non-intestinal infectious conditions"

Abstract:

Orally ingested probiotic micro-organisms do not exert health effects exclusively in the intestine. Some strains can alleviate or prevent bacterial, fungal or viral infections in other organs by stimulation of the immune system. By preservation or improvement of the barrier function of the intestinal mucosa, they may inhibit translocation of potential pathogens and thus prevent infections of the blood stream and other tissues and organs. Modulation of the intestinal microflora can affect the local microflora of the urogenital tract and possibly of the oral cavity. Finally, some strains of orally ingested bacteria reach target organs like the urogenital tract in a viable state; alternatively they can be applied locally.

Probiotic Bacteria

Despite the infection-preventing properties of probiotic bacteria, lactic acid bacteria have rarely been identified in infections of the blood stream, heart valves and other organs, usually only in patients with severe disease. It is the general opinion that in most cases the source of infection was the commensal microflora of the intestine or the oral cavity. Until now only one case of infection associated with administration of a probiotic strain has been published.

The most promising health-promoting effects have been seen in vaginosis, urinary tract infections, Helicobacter pylori gastritis and infections of the respiratory tract in children. More controlled clinical trials with sufficient numbers of participants are needed to determine the scientific basis for the use of probiotic bacteria in infections in locations of the body other than the intestine.

ME COMMENTS:

This study points out that probiotics also exert influence outside of the intestines.

ঔঌঔঌ

Probiotics instead of Antibiotics

In the journal *Trends Biotechnol.* 2003; 21(5):217-23 (ISSN: 0167-7799)

JR Tagg, et al., studied...

"Bacterial replacement therapy: adapting 'germ warfare' to infection prevention"

and found...

The individual bacterial members of our indigeneous microbiota are actively engaged in an on-going battle to prevent colonisation and overgrowth of their terrain by competing microbes, some of which might have pathogenic potential for the host. Humans have long attempted to intervene in these bacterial interactions. Ingestion of probiotic bacteria, particularly lactobacilli, is commonly practiced to promote well-balanced intestinal microflora. **As bacterial resistance to antimicrobials has increased, so too has research into colonisation of human tissues with specific effector strains capable of out-competing known bacterial pathogens.** Recent progress is particularly evident in the application of avirulent Streptococcus mutans to the control of dental caries, alpha hemolytic streptococci to reduction of otitis media recurrences and Streptococcus salivarius to streptococcal pharyngitis prevention.

ME COMMENTS:

This study follows the theory that instead of treating bacterial infections with antibiotics let us look at using probiotics. By increasing the number of friendly bacteria, it will be difficult for the pathogenic bacteria to survive.

ଓଃଓଃ

Probiotics and Urinary Tract Infection

In the journal *Infect Immun.* 1985 January; 47(1): 84–89.

R C Chan, et al., studied

"Competitive exclusion of uropathogens from human uroepithelial cells by Lactobacillus whole cells and cell wall fragments."

and found...

Previous studies have shown that indigenous bacteria isolated from cervical, vaginal, and urethral surfaces of healthy women are able to adhere to human uroepithelial cells in vitro. Furthermore, these organisms were found to block the adherence of uropathogenic bacteria to uroepithelial cells from women with and without a history of urinary tract infections. In the present study, complete or partial inhibition of the adherence of gram-negative uropathogens was achieved by preincubating the uroepithelial cells with bacterial cell wall fragments isolated from a Lactobacillus strain. Competitive exclusion was most effective with whole viable cells and less effective with cell wall fragments obtained by sonication, extraction with sodium dodecyl sulfate, and treatment with sodium dodecyl sulfate and acid. Analysis of the Lactobacillus cell wall preparations suggested that lipoteichoic acid was responsible for the adherence of the Lactobacillus cells to uroepithelial cells but that steric hindrance was the major factor in preventing the adherence of uropathogens.

This conclusion was also supported by blockage studies with reconstituted lipoteichoic acid-peptidoglycan, which was more effective at blocking adherence than lipoteichoic acid or peptidoglycan alone. **The results suggest that the normal flora of the urinary tract may be used to protect against the attachment of uropathogens to the surfaces of uroepithelial cells.** The long-term implications of these findings may lead to alternative methods for the management and prevention of recurrent urinary tract infections in females.

ME COMMENTS:

A theory that friendly bacteria can adhere to the surface which lines the vaginal, urethral and cervical walls thereby protecting us from pathogens.

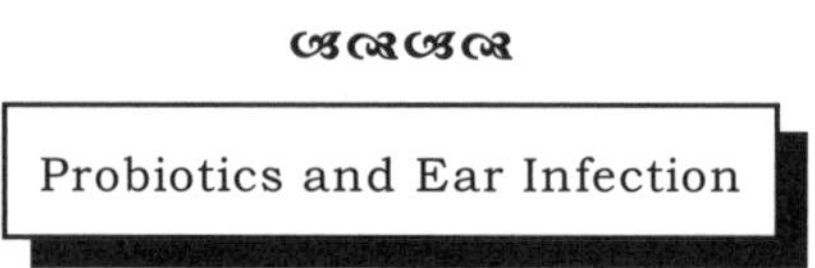

Probiotics and Ear Infection

In the *British Medical Journal* 2001;322:210 (27 January)

Kristian Roos, et al., studied...

"Effect of recolonisation with 'interfering' alpha streptococci on recurrences of acute and secretory otitis media in children: randomised placebo controlled trial"

Objective: To study the effect of recolonisation with alpha streptococci with the ability to inhibit the growth of otopathogens ("interfering" activity) on the recurrence of acute otitis media in susceptible children and the effect on the frequency of secretory otitis media.

Design: Double blind, randomised, placebo controlled study.

Setting: Ear, nose, and throat clinic with three doctors.

Participants: 130 children prone to otitis media aged between 6 months and 6 years, 108 of whom were eligible and followed for 3 months.

Main outcome measures: Recurrence of otitis media during follow up and a normal tympanic membrane at the last valid visit.

Interventions: Children with no recurrences during the last month received phenoxymethylpenicillin (n=22), and those with a recurrence within 1 month received amoxicillin clavulanic acid (n=86), both twice daily for 10 days. These were followed by a streptococcal or placebo solution sprayed into the nose for a further 10 days. At day 60 the same spray was started for another 10 days.

Results: At 3 months 22 children (42%) given the streptococcal spray were healthy and had a normal tympanic membrane compared with 12 (22%) of those given placebo. This difference was shown separately for recurrences of both acute otitis media and secretory otitis media.

Conclusions: Selected bacteria with the ability to inhibit the growth of common otopathogens can be used to protect against recurrent acute otitis media and secretory otitis media in children.

ME COMMENTS:

More scientific research validating the use of specific probiotics to treat ear infections.

ଓଷଓଷ

Probiotics and Vaginal and Bladder Infections

"Contemporary Issues in Ob/Gyn & Women's Health" *Medscape General Medicine.* 2004;6(1):e38. ©2004 Medscape

Dr. Gregor Reid, et al. studied...

"The Rationale for Probiotics in Female Urogenital Healthcare"

and found...

Urogenital infections are a major reason that women visit their family physician and are referred to gastroenterology, gynecology, urology, and infectious disease specialists. The association between abnormal vaginal microbiota and increased risk for sexually transmitted infections, bladder and vaginal infections per se, and a higher rate of preterm labor indicate the need to better understand and manage urogenital health. The concept of probiotics arose from the realization that humans are inhabited with microbes from birth and that these organisms play a role in preventing disease. Defined as "live microorganisms, which when administered in adequate amounts confer a health benefit on the host," probiotic strains have already been shown to effectively prevent diarrhea and to hold potential in preventing and treating tonsillitis, caries, renal calculi, and respiratory infections. **This review provides a rationale for the use of probiotics in maintaining female vaginal and bladder health and as a treatment option for recurrent bacterial vaginosis, urinary tract infection, yeast vaginitis, and sexually transmitted infections.** We consider only probiotic strains that fulfill the United Nations/World Health Organization Guidelines for Probiotics in being fully characterized and clinically documented through scientific investigations describing known or presumed mechanisms of action. Although medical practitioners as yet are unable to access these probiotic strains, an awareness of recent and ongoing research for probiotics is important, as results are encouraging. **The concept of probiotic therapy is familiar to many consumers and although it has historically lacked credibility in the medical community, perceptions are changing.**

ME COMMENTS:

The medical community is finally starting to catch up with the natural pharmaceutical community. However, they have a long way to go.

ઉଷ ઉଷ

Probiotics and Allergy

In the journal *Immunology and Allergy Clinics of North America* 01-NOV-2004; 24(4): 739-52, viii

MA Kalliomäki, et. al., studied...

"Probiotics and down-regulation of the allergic response."

Abstract:

The first clinical trials with probiotics, especially in the treatment of atopic eczema, have yielded encouraging results. **Experimental studies have found that probiotics exert strain-specific effects in the intestinal lumen and on epithelial cells and immune cells with anti-allergic potential.** These effects include enhancement in antigen degradation and gut barrier function and induction of regulatory and proinflammatory immune responses, the latter of which occurs more likely beyond the intestinal epithelium. Future studies should address more accurately how these and other possible mechanisms operate in the complex gastrointestinal macroenvironment in vivo and how these mechanisms are related to the clinical effects in a dose--dependent manner.

❧❧❧❧

Probiotics and NEC

In the journal *Clinics in Perinatology* 01-MAR-2004; 31(1): 157-67

KM Reber, et al., studied...

"Necrotizing enterocolitis: preventative strategies."

Abstract:

Necrotizing enterocolitis (NEC) remains a major cause of morbidity and mortality in premature infants. Although the pathogenesis of NEC is unclear, prevention strategies have been developed based on clinical observations and epidemiologic and experimental data. Most current strategies have centered on feeding practices (e.g., institution of feeds, advancement of feeds, composition of feeds, and standardization of feeding practices). **Emerging strategies [to lower the incidence of Necrotizing enterocolitis] include amino acid supplementation, the use of platelet-activating factor(PAF) antagonists or PAF-acetylhydrolase administration, polyunsaturated fatty acid administration, epidermal growth factor administration, and the use of pre- and probiotics.**

ଓଃଓଃ

Probiotics and NEC

In the journal *Clinics in Perinatology* 01-SEP-2004; 31(3): 489-500

C. Hammerman, et al., studied...

"Germ warfare: probiotics in defense of the premature gut."

Abstract:

The potential benefits of a predominantly lactic acid bacterial flora include an improved balance of gut microbial ecology and decreased susceptibility of the gut mucosa to bacterial translocation via adherence to the intestinal mucosa, strengthening mucosal barrier function. These properties should be especially beneficial to the premature neonate with (1) delayed establishment of normal flora, increasing the potential for proliferation of pathogenic bacteria and (2) immature development of the intestinal mucosa, rendering it more susceptible to the translocation of these pathogenic bacteria and leading to extra-intestinal spread and systemic disease. **Early probiotic supplementation in preterm infants is theoretically sound and associated with minimal risk. Clinical data remain preliminary but are supportive of a reduction in feeding intolerance and NEC in this high-risk group.**

ME COMMENTS:

NEC is a serious GI disease that affects mostly premature babies. It is six to ten times more likely to occur in bottle fed babies. It would seem to make more sense to give the mother probiotics and prebiotics so that she can transfer the extra friendly bacteria to her baby via breast milk.

ଓଷଓଷ

Probiotics and UTI

In the journal *Infectious Disease Clinics of North America* 01-JUN-2003; 17(2): 457-71

A. Stapleton studied...

"Novel approaches to prevention of urinary tract infections."

Abstract:

Urinary tract infections are common clinical entities occurring in a variety of patient groups, most frequently caused by uropathogenic E. coli. **Novel methods of preventing UTI currently under development are focused on three key approaches: (1) use of cranberry products, (2) restoration of the normal flora using Lactobacillus-based probiotic preparations, and (3) vaccine development.** Although promising studies in each of these areas have been published or are ongoing, additional properly designed and powered clinical studies based on solid scientific evidence are needed.

ME COMMENTS:

The scientists keep calling for more and more studies on probiotics, but keep prescribing more and more antibiotics for urinary tract infections, causing increased resistance in various strains of pathogenic bacteria.

ଓଷଓଷ

Probiotics and AAD

In the *British Medical Journal* 2002;324:1361 (8 June)

Aloysius L D'Souza, et al., studied

"Probiotics in prevention of antibiotic associated diarrhoea [AAD]: meta-analysis"

Objective: To evaluate efficacy of probiotics in prevention and treatment of diarrhoea associated with the use of antibiotics.

Design: Meta-analysis; outcome data (proportion of patients not getting diarrhoea) were analysed, pooled, and compared to determine odds ratios in treated and control groups.

Identification: Studies identified by searching Medline between 1966 and 2000 and the Cochrane Library.

Studies reviewed Nine randomised, double blind, placebo controlled trials of probiotics.

Results: Two of the nine studies investigated the effects of probiotics in children. Four trials used a yeast (Saccharomyces boulardii), four used lactobacilli, and one used a strain of enterococcus that produced lactic acid. Three trials used a combination of probiotic strains of bacteria. In all nine trials, the probiotics were given in combination with antibiotics and the control groups received placebo and antibiotics. The odds ratio in favour of active treatment over placebo in preventing diarrhoea associated with antibiotics was 0.39 (95% confidence interval 0.25 to 0.62; P<0.001) for the yeast and 0.34 (0.19 to 0.61; P<0.01 for lactobacilli. The combined odds ratio was 0.37 (0.26 to 0.53; P<0.001) in favour of active treatment over placebo.

Conclusions: The meta-analysis suggests that probiotics can be used to prevent antibiotic associated diarrhoea and that S boulardii and lactobacilli have the potential to be used in this situation. The efficacy of probiotics in treating antibiotic associated diarrhoea remains to be proved. A further large trial in which probiotics are used as preventive agents should look at the costs of and need for routine use of these agents.

Probiotics and AAD

In the *British Medical Journal* 2002;324:1345-1346 (8 June)

Frédéric Barbut, head of infection control, studied

"Managing antibiotic associated diarrhoea - Probiotics may help in prevention"

Diarrhoea is a common adverse effect of antibiotic treatments. Antibiotic associated diarrhoea occurs in about 5-30% of patients either early during antibiotic therapy or up to two months after the end of the treatment.1-3 The frequency of antibiotic associated diarrhoea depends on the definition of diarrhoea, the inciting antimicrobial agents, and host factors.

Almost all antibiotics, particularly those that act on anaerobes, can cause diarrhoea, but the risk is higher with aminopenicillins, a combination of aminopenicillins and clavulanate, cephalosporins, and clindamycin. Host factors for antibiotic associated diarrhoea include age over 65, immunosuppression, being in an intensive care unit, and prolonged hospitalisation.

Clinical presentations of antibiotic associated diarrhoea range from mild diarrhoea to fulminant pseudomembranous colitis. The latter is characterised by a watery diarrhoea, fever (in 80% of cases), leucocytosis (80%), and the presence of pseudomembranes on endoscopic examination. Severe complications include toxic megacolon, perforation, and shock.

Antibiotic associated diarrhoea results from disruption of the normal microflora of the gut by antibiotics....

...Managing the diarrhoea depends on the clinical presentation and the inciting agent.7-10 In mild to moderate diarrhoea conventional measures include rehydration or discontinuation of the inciting agent or its replacement by an antibiotic with a lower risk of inducing diarrhoea, such as quinolones, co-trimoxazole, or aminoglycosides. In 22% of cases of diarrhoea related to C difficile, withdrawal of the inciting agent will lead to resolution of clinical signs in three days.

Probiotic Bacteria

In cases of severe or persistent antibiotic associated diarrhoea, the challenge is to identify C difficile associated infections since this is the most common identifiable and treatable pathogen. Diagnosis relies on detecting toxins A or B in stools. Tissue culture assay is the gold standard, although it is time consuming. Enzyme immunoassays for toxins A or B have a good specificity but a false negative rate of 10-20%....

...As antibiotic associated diarrhoea mostly results from a disequilibrium of the normal intestinal flora, research has focused on the benefits of administering living organisms (probiotics or biotherapeutic agents) to restore the normal flora. Numerous probiotics such as Lactobacillus acidophilus, L casei GG, L bulgaricus, Bifidobacterium bifidum, B longum, Enterococcus faecium, Streptococcus thermophilus, or Saccharomyces boulardii have been tested for the treatment and prevention of antibiotic associated diarrhoea. The benefits of probiotics are unproved as few have been evaluated in double blind placebo controlled studies. The results of the small and open trials of treatment are conflicting.

Most studies with probiotics have assessed their use in preventing antibiotic associated diarrhoea. In this issue D'Souza et al report a meta-analysis of nine randomised double blind trials comparing probiotics with placebo in the prevention of diarrhoea. Among these studies, four trials were used S boulardii and five Lactobacillus. Their results suggest that probiotics are useful in prevention. The expected advantages of probiotics include ease of administration, cost effectiveness, and relative lack of side effects. However, several cases of bacteraemia with S boulardii have been reported, which should prompt caution in the use of this yeast in immunosuppressed patients or patients with underlying disorders.

The key measure for preventing antibiotic associated diarrhoea, however, is to limit antibiotic use. Probiotics have proved useful in preventing diarrhoea, but the number of clinical trials is limited and further controlled trials using different probiotics are needed. In the case of C difficile related diarrhoea hygiene measures (single rooms, use of gloves, and handwashing) should be systematically associated with treatment in order to prevent transmission and dissemination of this nosocomial bacteria.

ME COMMENTS:

Dr. Frédéric Barbut makes a most important point. The best treatment for AAD is to limit antibiotic use. We know that antibiotics are prescribed beyond their usefulness. The goal is not to give probiotics to treat AAD, but to limit the use of antibiotics.

☙❧☙❧

Probiotics
Treatment for AAD and Clostridium difficile

In the British Medical Journal 2002 324: 1361

Aloysius L D'Souza, et al., studied

"Probiotics in prevention of antibiotic associated diarrhoea: meta-analysis"

A systematic review of nine trials by D'Souza and colleagues finds that probiotics can be used to prevent antibiotic associated diarrhoea, but that their efficacy in treating the condition remains to be proved. Probiotics are becoming increasingly available as capsules and dairy based food supplements and have few side effects. **The authors say that doctors should consider using them to prevent antibiotic associated diarrhoea and infection with Clostridium difficile.**

ME COMMENTS:

C-Diff used to be a problem only for the elderly, severely immune compromised persons and people on antibiotics, but no longer. The abuse of antibiotics has resulted in this deadly bacteria being found in healthy individuals. This bacteria C-Diff has become a threat in hospitals and nursing homes. Last year over 100 deaths in a hospital in Quebec, Canada were attributed to it. According to a CDC report in December 2005 recent cases in four states show it is appearing more often in healthy people who have not been admitted to healthcare facilities or even taken antibiotics. The CDC report focused on 33 cases reported since 2003. Twenty three involved otherwise healthy people in the Philadelphia area who were not admitted to the hospital within three months of illness. Ten more were otherwise healthy pregnant women or women who had recently given birth and had brief hospital stays. One of the 33 patients who died was a 31 year old Pennsylvania woman, who was 14 weeks pregnant with twins when she first went to the ER with symptoms. Despite treatment with antibiotics, considered effective against C-Diff, she miscarried and subsequently died. She had been treated about 3 months earlier for an urinary tract infection with an antibiotic.

These findings should make physicians more wary when they prescribe antibiotics and consider using probiotics as a first line of defense.

ઙ૨ઙ૨

Probiotics and H pylori

In the journal *Digestive Diseases and Sciences.* 2004; 49(7-8):1095-102

KC Johnson-Henry, et al., studied....

"Probiotics reduce bacterial colonization and gastric inflammation in H. pylori-infected mice."

Probiotics are characterized by their ability to interact with commensal microflora in the gastrointestinal tract to produce beneficial health effects. In vitro studies suggest that Lactobacillus species have the potential to suppress the growth of Helicobacter pylori. The goal of this study was to determine if pretreatment of mice with a commercial mixture of live probiotics (L. rhamnosus, strain R0011, and L. acidophilus, strain R0052) would suppress colonization of H. pylori, strain SS1. Thirty C57BL/6 female mice were divided into four groups: Group A was fed sterile water, group B received probiotics in sterile drinking water, group C was challenged orogastrically with H. pylori, and group D was pretreated with probiotics in drinking water prior to and following challenge with H. pylori. Rectal swabs, stomach homogenates, and luminal contents from ileum and colon were plated onto colistin nalidixic acid plates. Serial dilutions of stomach homogenates were plated onto H. pylori-sensitive agar plates and incubated under microaerophilic conditions. Tissue samples from the stomach were analyzed histologically to determine the degree of H. pylori colonization, mucosal inflammation, and epithelial cell apoptosis. Probiotics in drinking water did not affect the overall well-being of mice. Lactobacillus species were excreted in stools over the entire duration of treatment. Pretreatment with probiotics reduced the number of mice with H. pylori growth from stomach homgenates (100 to 50%; P = 0.02). The percentage of mice with moderate-severe H. pylori-induced inflammation in the gastric antrum was reduced with probiotic pretreatment (71 to 29%; P = 0.14). **However, pretreatment with probiotics did not prevent H. pylori-induced apoptosis in the gastric mucosa. This preparation of probiotics provided a safe and novel approach for reducing H. pylori colonization and bacterial-induced inflammation of mice.**

ଔଓଔଓ

Probiotics and Allergy

In the *Journal of Allergy and Clinical Immunology* 01-JUL-2005; 116(1): 31-7

S Rautava, et al., studied...

"New therapeutic strategy for combating the increasing burden of allergic disease: Probiotics-A Nutrition, Allergy, Mucosal Immunology and Intestinal Microbiota"

Abstract:

The dietary approach to reducing the risk of atopic diseases in infancy is evolving from passive allergen avoidance to active stimulation of the immature immune system, the aim of which is to support the establishment of tolerance. The intestinal mucosa and the mucosa-associated immune system are the primary loci of allergen contact and induction of immune responsiveness. In this review we discuss cross-talk between the intestinal microbiota and the host as it pertains to healthy immunologic maturation.

Understanding these complex phenomena provides the rationale for the use of probiotics in reducing the risk and nutritional management of atopic disease.

ଓଓଓଓ

Probiotics and breastfeeding

In the *Journal of Pediatrics*. 01-AUG-2005; 147(2): 186-91

M. Rinne, et al., studied...

"Effect of probiotics and breastfeeding on the bifidobacterium and lactobacillus/enterococcus microbiota and humoral immune responses."

Abstract:

OBJECTIVE: To assess impact of probiotics and breastfeeding on gut microecology. STUDY DESIGN: Mothers were randomized to receive placebo or Lactobacillus rhamnosus GG before delivery, with treatment of the infants after delivery. We assessed gut microbiota, humoral immune responses, and measured soluble cluster of differentiation 14 (sCD14) in colostrum in 96 infants. RESULTS: Fecal Bifidobacterium and Lactobacillus/ Enterococcus counts were higher in breastfed than formula-fed infants at 6 months; P <.0001 and P=.01, respectively. At 3 months, total number of immunoglobulin (Ig)G-secreting cells in breastfed infants supplemented with probiotics exceeded those in breastfed infants receiving placebo; P=.05, and their number correlated with concentration of sCD14 in colostrum. Total numbers of IgM-, IgA-, and IgG-secreting cells at 12 months were higher in infants breastfed exclusively for at least for 3 months and supplemented with probiotics as compared with breastfed infants receiving placebo; P=.005, P=.03 and P=.04, respectively. Again, sCD14 in colostrum correlated with numbers of IgM and IgA cells; P=.05 in both.

CONCLUSIONS: We found an interaction between probiotics and breastfeeding on number of Ig-secreting cells, suggesting

that probiotics during breastfeeding may positively influence gut immunity.

ME COMMENTS:

This study shows that probiotics taken by the nursing mother will increase the number of friendly bacteria in the baby.

ᏟᏡᏟᏡ

Probiotics and breastfeeding

In the *Journal of Allergy and Clinical Immunology* 2002; 109(1):119-21

S. Rautava, et. al., studied...

> **"Probiotics during pregnancy and breastfeeding might confer immunomodulatory protection against atopic disease in the infant."**

The prevalence of atopic diseases is increasing throughout the Western world, and means of primary prevention are needed to reverse this trend. The role of breast-feeding, the best source of infant nutrition, in protection against atopic disease remains elusive. In this double-blinded, placebo-controlled study of 62 mother-infant pairs, it is shown that administering probiotics to the pregnant and lactating mother increased the immunoprotective potential of breast milk, as assessed by the amount of anti-inflammatory transforming growth factor beta2 (TGF-beta2) in the milk (2885 pg/mL [95% CI, 1624-4146] in mothers receiving probiotics vs 1340 pg/mL [95% CI, 978-1702] in mothers receiving placebo; P =.018). The risk of developing atopic eczema during the first 2 years of life in infants whose mothers received probiotics was significantly reduced in comparison with that in infants whose mothers received placebo (15% and 47%, respectively; relative risk, 0.32 [95% CI, 0.12-0.85]; P =.0098). Maternal atopy was a clear risk factor for atopic eczema in the infant. The infants most likely to benefit from maternal probiotic supplementation were those with an elevated cord blood IgE concentration.

Administering probiotics during pregnancy and breast-feeding thus offers a safe and effective mode of promoting the immunoprotective potential of breast-feeding and provides protection against atopic eczema during the first 2 years of life.

ଓଓଓଓ

Probiotics and SCFAs

In the *American Journal of Clinical Nutrition*, 01-JUL-2004; 80(1): 89-94

JA Vogt, et al., studied...

"L-Rhamnose increases serum propionate in humans."

Abstract:

BACKGROUND: Acetic and propionic acids are produced by colonic bacterial fermentation of unabsorbed carbohydrates and are absorbed into the portal circulation. From there, they travel to the liver, where acetate is a lipogenic substrate and propionate can inhibit lipogenesis. The extent to which peripheral blood short--chain fatty acid concentrations reflect differences in colonic fermentation is uncertain. The unabsorbed sugar lactulose produces mainly acetate when fermented in vitro, whereas L-rhamnose yields propionate. OBJECTIVE: The objective of the study was to ascertain whether ingestion of L-rhamnose and lactulose would have different acute effects on peripheral acetate and propionate concentrations and on breath hydrogen and methane concentrations. DESIGN: Twenty-two subjects were fed 25 g L-rhamnose, lactulose, or glucose on 3 separate occasions in a randomized crossover design. Blood and breath samples were collected hourly for 12 h. RESULTS: Serum propionate was significantly higher with ingestion of L-rhamnose than with that of lactulose or glucose ($P < 0.001$). The area under the curve for serum acetate was significantly higher with ingestion of lactulose than with that of glucose ($P < 0.03$). The ratio of serum acetate to propionate was significantly higher with ingestion of lactulose than with that of glucose or L-rhamnose ($P < 0.01$). Breath hydrogen was significantly higher with ingestion of lactulose than with that of L-rhamnose or glucose ($P < 0.0001$).

CONCLUSIONS: The selective increases in serum acetate and propionate concentrations in humans were obtained by feeding specific fermentable substrates. Presumably, these changes in serum concentrations reflect changes in colonic production. Selective alteration of colonic fermentation products could yield a new mechanism for modifying blood lipids.

ଔଓଔଓ

Friendly Bacteria and Friendly Yeast in Place of Antibiotics

In the journal *Communicable Diseases Intelligence*, 01-JAN-2003; 27 Suppl: S143-6

CF Carson, et al., studied...

"Non-antibiotic therapies for infectious diseases."

Abstract:

The emergence of multiple antibiotic resistant organisms in the general community is a potentially serious threat to public health. The emergence of antibiotic resistance has not yet prompted a radical revision of antibiotic utilisation. Instead it has prompted the development of additional antibiotics. Unfortunately, this does not relieve the underlying selection pressure that drives the development of resistance. **A paradigm shift in the treatment of infectious disease is necessary to prevent antibiotics becoming obsolete and, where appropriate, alternatives to antibiotics ought to be considered.** There are already several non-antibiotic approaches to the treatment and prevention of infection including probiotics, phages and phytomedicines. There is some evidence that probiotics such as Lactobacillus spp. or Saccharomyces boulardii are useful in the prevention and treatment of diarrhoea, including Clostridium difficile-associated diarrhoea that can be difficult to treat and recurs frequently. Bacteriophages have received renewed attention for the control of both staphylococcal and gastrointestinal infections. Phytomedicines that have been utilised in the treatment of infections include artesunate for malaria, tea tree oil for skin infections, honey for wound infections, mastic gum for Helicobacter pylori gastric ulcers and cranberry juice for urinary tract infections. Many infections may prove amenable to safe and effective treatment with non-antibiotics.

ME COMMENTS:

There are many non-antibiotic, alternative treatments for infections (i.e., probiotics), to be found by unlocking nature's pharmacy to solve the problem of antibiotic abuse.

ଔଊଔଊ

SACCROMYCES BOULLARDII
Friendly Yeast

Saccharomyces boulardii is a nonpathogenic, non-colonizing "friendly yeast" that is recognized to have probiotic effectiveness when used alone or in combination with other probiotic bacteria.

To be effective a probiotic must:

- Be safe (e.g. of human origin and non-pathogenic)
- Be resistant to technologic processes and exert minimal sensory influence on the probiotic food
- Be resistant to passage through the gastrointestinal tract, not broken down by gastric acidity and bile acids
- Adhere to the gut epithelial tissue and possess growth capability
- Provide health benefits

Saccromyces Boullardii is a unique probiotic in that it is known to survive gastric acidity. It is not adversely affected or inhibited by antibiotics and does not alter or adversely affect the friendly bacteria in the intestines. It can be taken along with probiotic bacterial organisms (see glossary for list). However, Sacromyces boullardii is destroyed by anti-fungals, i.e., Nystatin Diflucan, Lamasil, etc. Thus it must be taken at a different time than an anti-fungal.

Sacromyces boullardii, although it is classified as a yeast, is not related to the Candida species, a pathogenic yeast which causes vaginal and oral yeast infections, etc.

Saccromyces boullardii is prescribed in a lyophilized (freeze-dried) form and acts as a biotherapeutic agent. Controlled clinical trials have demonstrated the efficacy of Saccromyces boullardii for preventing or treating several intestinal disorders including:

Saccromyces Boullardii

- AAD - antibiotic associated diarrhea
- C difficile
- enterocolopathies
- acute gastroenteritis
- traveler's diarrhea
- TEN diarrhea
- AIDS diarrhea
- IBS
- Chronic Inflammatory Bowel Disease

After oral administration of lyophilized Saccromyces boullardii steady-state concentrations of viable yeast cells are achieved within a mean of 3 days, and the cells are cleared from the stools within 2 to 5 days after discontinuation. Thus, Saccromyces boullardii rapidly reaches the gastrointestinal (GI) tract in high concentrations and remains in a viable form throughout the bowel. Saccromyces boullardii exerts several beneficial effects on the host GI tract including protective effects against:

- enteric pathogens such as Vibrio cholerae
- C difficile
- Escherichia coli
- lysis of enterotoxins and their binding to intestinal receptors
- stimulation of immune host defenses
- inhibition of the inflammatory response induced by enterotoxins, and
- enhancement of trophic factors such as brush border membrane enzymes and nutrient transporters

According to these pharmacological and clinical data, Saccromyces boullardii is a biotherapeutic medication, clearly distinct from probiotic bacteria which contain various species of microorganisms and prebiotic substances which feed the friendly bacteria.

Saccromyces boullardii has an effect on the metabolism of short-chain fatty acids (SCFAs). SCFAs are among the most important metabolites produced by the friendly bacteria. They play a major role in colonic reabsorption of water and electrolytes. In a porcine model of bacterial ecosystem, administration of Saccromyces boullardii was able to restore production of SCFAs to normal levels which had been depressed by the decrease of bacterial mass due to Clindamycin treatment.

This can play a role in acute gastroenteritis and explain, in part, the antidiarrheal effect of Saccromyces boullardii. SCFAs are decreased in relation to microflora alterations in antibiotic-associated diarrhea and diarrhea occurring during continuous enteral feeding.

The following scientific studies document the evidence based approach to using Saccromyces boullardii for many conditions.

Saccromyces Boullardii and Diarrhea

In the journal *Digestive Diseases and Sciences*, 01-NOV-2005; 50(11): 2183-90

P. Girard, et al., studied...

"Saccharomyces boulardii inhibits water and electrolytes changes induced by castor oil in the rat colon."

Abstract:

The biotherapeutic agent Saccharomyces boulardii has been shown to inhibit castor oil-induced diarrhoea in rats. The present study investigated the mechanism(s) of this antidiarrhoeal effect in terms of water and electrolyte (sodium, potassium and chloride) changes using two rat models. A single oral dose of S. boulardii of up to 12 x 10(10) CFU/kg of viable cells did not inhibit castor oil-induced fluid secretion in the enteropooling model. However, the yeast dose dependently reduced castor oil induced fluid secretion into the colon, with a significant protection at 12 x 10(10) CFU/kg. In this model, castor oil reversed net sodium and chloride absorption into net secretion, and increased net potassium secretion into the lumen. Single pre-treatment with S. boulardii at 4 and 12 x 10(10) CFU/kg dose dependently decreased these electrolyte changes.

In conclusion, S. boulardii possesses potent anti-secretory properties versus water and electrolyte secretion induced by castor oil in the rat colon.

ᏒᏒ

Saccromyces Boullardii vs. Probiotic Bacteria

In the journal *British Poultry Science,* 01-AUG-2005; 46(4): 494-7

JR Gil de los Santos, et al., studied...

"Bacillus cereus var. toyoii and saccharomyces boulardii increased feed efficiency in broilers infected with Salmonella enteritidis."

Abstract:

1. The effect on feed efficiency of two probiotics, one prepared with Saccharomyces boulardii and the other with Bacillus cereus var. toyoii, was tested in broilers infected with Salmonella enteritidis. 2. One-day-old chicks were divided at random into three groups and fed commercial feed devoid of antibiotics: group 1 was fed with non-supplemented feed, group 2 was supplemented with S. boulardii and group 3 with B. cereus. At 14 d of age the animals were challenged by the oral route with 1 x 10(7) viable S. enteritidis. 3. At d 47, average live weights were: group 1, 1.77 kg, group 2, 1.89 kg and group 3, 2.06 kg, and were significantly different. Feed conversion rates were 2.61 for group 1, 2.35 for group 2 and 2.30 for group 3. 4. **We conclude that both probiotics improved feed efficiency in broilers.**

ଓଌଓଌ

Saccromyces Boullardii and Travelers Diarrhea

In the *World Journal of Gastroenterology*, 01-AUG-2003; 9(8): 1832-3

F. Mansour-Ghanaei, et al., studied...

"Efficacy of saccharomyces boulardii with antibiotics in acute amoebiasis."

Abstract:

AIM: To compare the efficacy of antibiotics therapy alone with antibiotics and saccharomyces boulardii in treatment of acute amebiasis. METHODS: In a double blind, random clinical trial on patients with acute intestinal amoebiasis, 57 adult patients with acute amoebiasis, diagnosed with clinical manifestations (acute mucous bloody diarrhea) and amebic trophozoites engulfing RBCs found in stool were enrolled in the study...

...CONCLUSION: Adding saccharomyces boulardii to antibiotics in the treatment of acute amebiasis seems to decrease the duration of clinical symptoms and cyst passage.

ME COMMENTS:

Amebiasis is the leading cause of traveler's diarrhea.

Saccromyces Boullardii and AAD

In the journal *Alimentary Pharmacology and Therapeutics*, 1-SEP-2005; 22(5): 365-72

H. Szajewska, et al., studied...

"Meta-analysis: non-pathogenic yeast Saccharomyces boulardii in the prevention of antibiotic-associated diarrhoea."

Abstract:

BACKGROUND: Antibiotic-associated diarrhoea occurs in up to 30% of patients who receive antibiotics but can be prevented with probiotics. AIM: To systematically evaluate the effectiveness of Saccharomyces boulardii in preventing antibiotic-associated diarrhoea in children and adults...

...CONCLUSIONS: A meta-analysis of data from five randomized-controlled trials showed that S. boulardii is moderately effective in preventing antibiotic-associated diarrhoea in children and adults treated with antibiotics for any reason (mainly respiratory tract infections). For every 10 patients receiving daily S. boulardii with antibiotics, one fewer will develop antibiotic-associated diarrhoea.

ME COMMENTS:

My clinical experience has shown that 7 out of 10 patients on antibiotics experience no diarrhea when treated along with SACCROMYCES boullardii. I recommend SACCROMYCES boullardii for everyone who is on antibiotics. Since SACCROMYCES boullardii is a friendly yeast it will not be destroyed by the antibiotics and can be taken at the same time.

Saccromyces Boullardii and Colitis

In the *Journal of the American Veterinary Medical Association*, 15-SEP-2005; 227(6): 954-9

AM Desrochers, et al., studied...

"Efficacy of Saccharomyces boulardii for treatment of horses with acute enterocolitis."

Abstract:

OBJECTIVE: To evaluate the viability of Saccharomyces boulardii after PO administration in clinically normal horses and its efficacy as a treatment for horses with acute enterocolitis...

...CONCLUSIONS AND CLINICAL RELEVANCE: Administration of S. boulardii may help decrease the severity and duration of clinical signs in horses with acute enterocolitis.

ME COMMENTS:

I have had the same results in clinical practice. SACCROMYCES boullardii has been an exceptional treatment for antibiotic associated diarrhea (AAD).

ꟹꟹꟹꟹ

Saccromyces Boullardii and Prevention of AAD

In the journal *Alimentary Pharmacology and Therapeutics*, 1-MAR-2005; 21(5): 583-90

M. Kotowska, et al., studied...

"Saccharomyces boulardii in the prevention of antibiotic-associated diarrhoea in children: a randomized double-blind placebo-controlled trial."

Abstract:

BACKGROUND: Co-treatment with Saccharomyces boulardii appears to lower the risk of antibiotic-associated diarrhoea in adults receiving broad-spectrum antibiotics. AIM: To determine whether S. boulardii prevents antibiotic-associated diarrhoea in children. METHODS: A total of 269 children (aged 6 months to 14 years) with otitis media and/or respiratory tract infections were enrolled in a double-blind, randomized placebo-controlled trial in which they received standard antibiotic treatment plus 250 mg of S. boulardii (experimental group, n = 132) or a placebo (control group, n = 137) orally twice daily for the duration of antibiotic treatment. Analyses were based on allocated treatment and included data from 246 children. RESULTS: Patients receiving S. boulardii had a lower prevalence of diarrhoea (> or =3 loose or watery stools/day for > or =48 h occurring during or up to 2 weeks after the antibiotic therapy) than those receiving placebo [nine of 119 (8%) vs. 29 of 127 (23%), relative risk: 0.3, 95% confidence interval: 0.2-0.7]. S. boulardii also reduced the risk of antibiotic-associated diarrhoea (diarrhoea caused by Clostridium difficile or otherwise unexplained diarrhoea) compared with placebo [four of 119 (3.4%) vs. 22 of 127 (17.3%), relative risk: 0.2; 95% confidence interval: 0.07-0.5]. No adverse events were observed.

CONCLUSION: This is the first randomized-controlled trial evidence that Saccromyces boullardii effectively reduces the risk of antibiotic-associated diarrhoea in children.

ME COMMENTS:

This is an important study, for it points out something I have been implementing in my clinical practice for quite a while. That is whenever I put someone on an antibiotic (this applies to adults as well as children) I also prescribe Saccromyces boullardii at the same time. Since Saccromyces boullardii is a "friendly yeast" it will not be affected by the antibiotic. Therefore, you can take them simultaneously.

In most European countries Saccromyces boullardii is only available by prescription. In the United States it is available over the counter.

଍଍଍଍

Saccromyces Boullardii and Antibiotics

In the *Journal of Tropical Pediatrics,* 01-AUG-2004; 50(4): 234-6

O Erdeve, et al., studied...

"The probiotic effect of Saccharomyces boulardii in a pediatric age group."

Abstract:

The aim of this study was to determine the efficacy of S. boulardii in diarrhea associated with commonly used antibiotics such as sulbactam-ampicillin (SAM) and azithromycin (AZT). Four hundred and sixty-six patients were assigned to four different groups as follows: group 1:117 patients receiving SAM alone; group 2:117 patients receiving SAM and S. boulardii, group 3:105 patients receiving AZT alone; group 4:127 patients receiving AZT and S. boulardii. Antibiotic-associated diarrhea was seen in 42 of the 222 patients (18.9 per cent) receiving an antibiotic without the probiotic, and in 14 of the 244 patients (5.7 per cent) who received both the probiotic and the antibiotic ($p < 0.05$). In the group receiving SAM where S. boulardii use was found to be significant, **the use of S. boulardii decreased the diarrhea rate** from 32.3 to 11.4 per cent in the 1-5 years age group ($p < 0.05$). **This is a pioneering study investigating combined antibiotic and probiotic use in pediatric diarrhea patients.**

ଔଓଔଓ

Saccromyces Boullardii and SCFAs

In the *World Journal of Gastroenterology* ISSN 1007-9327 wjg@wjgnet.com © 2005

Stephanie M Schneider, et al., studied ...

"Effects of Saccharomyces Boulardii on fecal short-chain fatty acids and microflora in patients on long-term total enteral nutrition"

Abstract

AIM: To assess the effects of Saccharomyces Boulardii on fecal flora and shortchain fatty acids (SCFA) in patients on long-term TEN (total enteral nutrition).

CONCLUSION: Saccromyces boullardii-induced increase of fecal SCFA concentrations (especially butyrate) may explain the preventive effects of this yeast on TEN-induced diarrhea.

DISCUSSION: *Saccromyces boullardii* is known to interact with the intestinal flora. Yeast proteins have been shown to neutralize cholera toxin and to repress *Clostridium difficile* toxins A and B;

Saccromyces boullardii also has an antagonistic effect on the growth of pathogenic microorganisms in the intestine. In our study, increased SCFA concentrations might explain the reported prevention by *Saccromyces boullardii* of TEN-induced diarrhea by an increased water and electrolyte absorption and by a reduction in colonic pH, even though it was not measured in the stool samples from our subjects....

...In conclusion, this study suggests one possible mechanism of action of the probiotic yeast *Saccromyces boullardii*, especially for its preventive effects in enteral nutrition-induced diarrhea. **It also supports its use [Saccromyces boullardii] especially in patients who have other risk factors, such as antibiotic intake.**

ЖЖЖЖ

Saccromyces Boullardii and Clostridium difficile disease

In the *Journal of the American Medical Association.* 1994 Jun 22-29;271(24):1913-8.

LV McFarland, et. al., studied...

"A randomized placebo-controlled trial of Saccharomyces boulardii in combination with standard antibiotics for Clostridium difficile disease."

OBJECTIVE--To determine the safety and efficacy of a new combination treatment for patients with Clostridium difficile-associated disease (CDD). The treatment combines the yeast Saccharomyces boulardii with an antibiotic (vancomycin hydrochloride or metronidazole).

DESIGN--A double-blind, randomized, placebo-controlled, parallel-group intervention study in patients with active CDD. Patients received standard antibiotics and Saccromyces boullardii or placebo for 4 weeks, and were followed up for an additional 4 weeks after therapy. Effectiveness was determined by comparing the recurrence of CDD in the two groups using multivariate analysis to control for other risk factors for CDD.

Saccromyces Boullardii

SETTING--National referral study of ambulatory or hospitalized patients from three main study coordinating centers.

PATIENTS--A total of 124 eligible consenting adult patients, including 64 who were enrolled with an initial episode of CDD, and 60 who had a history of at least one prior CDD episode. Patients who were immunosuppressed due to acquired immunodeficiency syndrome or cancer chemotherapy within 3 months were not eligible.

INTERVENTION--Treatment with oral S boulardii (1 g/d for 4 weeks) or placebo in combination with a standard antibiotic. MAIN OUTCOME MEASURE--Recurrence of active CDD.

RESULTS--A history of CDD episodes dramatically increased the likelihood of further recurrences. Multivariate analysis revealed that patients treated with S boulardii and standard antibiotics had a significantly lower relative risk (RR) of CDD recurrence (RR, 0.43; 95% confidence interval, 0.20 to 0.97) compared with placebo and standard antibiotics. The efficacy of S boulardii was significant (recurrence rate 34.6%, compared with 64.7% on placebo; P = .04) in patients with recurrent CDD, but not in patients with initial CDD (recurrence rate 19.3% compared with 24.2% on placebo; P = .86). There were no serious adverse reactions associated with Saccromyces boullardii.

CONCLUSIONS--The combination of standard antibiotics and Saccromyces boullardii was shown to be an effective and safe therapy for these patients with recurrent CDD; no benefit of Saccromyces boullardii was demonstrated for those with an initial episode of CDD.

Saccromyces Boullardii and By-Pass Surgery

In the journal *Gut* 1999;45:89-96

N. Butsa, et al., studied...

"Saccharomyces boulardii upgrades cellular adaptation after proximal enterectomy in rats J-P"

BACKGROUND---Saccharomyces boulardii is a non-pathogenic yeast which exerts trophic effects on human and rat small intestinal mucosa.

AIMS---To examine the effects of Saccromyces boullardii on ileal adaptation after proximal enterectomy in rats.

METHODS---Wistar rats, aged eight weeks, underwent 60% proximal resection or transection and received by orogastric intubation either 1 mg/g body wt per day lyophilised Saccromyces boullardii or the vehicle for seven days. The effects on ileal mucosal adaptation were assessed eight days after surgery.

RESULTS---Compared with transection, resection resulted in mucosal hyperplasia with significant decreases in the specific and total activities of sucrase, lactase, and maltase. Treatment of resected animals with Saccromyces boullardii had no effect on mucosal hyperplasia but did upgrade disaccharidase activities to the levels of the transected group. Enzyme stimulation by Saccromyces boullardii was associated with significant increases in diamine oxidase activity and mucosal polyamine concentrations. Likewise, sodium dependent D-glucose uptake by brush border membrane vesicles, measured as a function of time and glucose concentration in the incubation medium, was significantly ($p<0.05$) increased by 81% and three times respectively in the resected group treated with Saccromyces boullardii. In agreement with this, expression of the sodium/glucose cotransporter-1 in brush border membranes of resected rats treated with Saccromyces boullardii was enhanced twofold compared with resected controls.

CONCLUSION---Oral administration of Saccromyces boullardii soon after proximal enterectomy improves functional adaptation of the remnant ileum.

ME COMMENTS:

By-pass surgery is becoming more and more common. One of the major side effects of by-pass surgery is dumping syndrome, a process where fluid loss from the intestine leads to severe and uncontrollable diarrhea. This study points out that Saccromyces boullardii may be helpful, in by-pass patients, to prevent fluid loss.

ઌઌઌઌ

PREBIOTICS

Prebiotics are nondigestible food ingredients that beneficially affect the host by selectively stimulating the growth and activity of a number of bacteria in the colon. In order to be effective, prebiotics must avoid digestion in the upper gastrointestinal (GI) tract and be used by a limited number of the microorganisms comprising the colonic microflora. Prebiotics are principally oligosaccharides. They mainly stimulate the growth of bifidobacteria and to a lesser degree lactobacteria.

The oligosaccharides escape digestion in the upper GI tract because they have bonds which cannot be broken down by human saliva or stomach enzymes. However, the friendly bacteria in the colon, both endogenous and exogenous, have the enzymes necessary to break down the bonds.

Oligosaccharides are among the most common food substances that qualify as prebiotics. The most studied of them is fructooligosaccharide (FOS), and to a lesser extent mannanoligosaccharide (MOS) and galactooligosaccharide (GOS).

Fructooligosaccharide or FOS typically refers to short-chain oligosaccharides comprised of D-fructose and D-glucose, containing from three to five monosaccharide units. FOS, also called neosugar and short-chain FOS (sc FOS), is produced commercially from sucrose, using a fungal fructosyltransferase enzyme. FOS is resistant to digestion in the upper gastrointestinal tract. It acts to stimulate the growth of bifidobacterium species in the large intestine.

FOS passes through the GI tract with minimal problems. It is of interest that the upper digestive system does not metabolize FOS, rather, it reaches the lower intestine intact, where it is devoured by the friendly bacteria, without significantly enhancing any unfriendly bacteria. These properties make FOS extremely beneficial in treating a variety of digestive problems.

Prebiotics

Since humans cannot digest FOS, you might think there is no caloric component yet, in a unique, round-about way, there is. Beneficial bacteria, such as bifidobacteria, consume FOS. The by-product of this FOS feast are short chain fatty acids (SCFAs). These fatty acids are absorbed by the wall of the large intestine and used for energy. The human body does not consume the FOS directly, but via their by-products - SCFAs. Without bifidobacteria, we would never get any calories from FOS. By this circuitous route, FOS contributes only approximately 1.5 calories per gram to the body. Digestible carbohydrates give the body four calories per gram. In order to get the benefit from friendly bacteria, one cannot merely take them and assume that they will thrive in the GI tract, where survival of the fittest is the rule. This is where FOS comes in. FOS selectively feeds the friendly bacteria helping them multiply.

Scientific studies show that oligosaccharides can:

- Selectively feed and encourage the growth of friendly bacteria such as bifidobacteria
- Reduce the growth of unfriendly bacteria and the putrefactive substances they produce in the digestive tract
- Lower blood cholesterol and triglyceride levels
- Improve the taste, texture and health benefits of a wide variety of foods
- Help diabetics lower blood sugar levels
- Increase absorption of minerals (calcium, magnesium and iron)
- Treat constipation
- Treat the diarrhea even that caused by Clostridium difficile
- Attach and destroy the cell membrane of pathogenic bacteria
- Provide approximately 1.5 calories per gram, less than one-half the caloric content of digestible carbohydrates (4 calories per gram)

Mannanoligosaccharide (MOS) passes through the GI tract with minimal problems. It is of interest that the digestive system does not break down MOS in the same way as FOS. Rather, it reaches the lower intestine intact where it attaches to the pathogenic bacteria causing the cell walls to rupture. These properties make MOS extremely beneficial in treating a variety of digestive problems. Studies have shown in some instances that MOS can be a substitute for antibiotics against the pathogenic bacteria which originate in the large intestine.

Oligosaccharides (i.e. FOS, MOS, GOS etc.) increase friendly bacteria levels by feeding the friendly bacteria. In order to have the highest number of friendly bacteria, prebiotics should be taken along with probiotics.

The following scientific studies document the evidence based approach to using prebiotics for many conditions.

FOS
Aids digestion, increases calcium and magnesium absorption.

In the journal *Biofactors* - 01-JAN-2004; 21(1-4): 89-94

T. Tokunaga, studied...

"Novel physiological function of fructooligosaccharides."

Abstract:

Two key properties of short chain fructooligosaccharides (sc-FOS) which lead to physiological functions are indigestibility in the small intestine and fermentability in the colon. Sc-FOS is converted into short chain fatty acids (SCFAs) by intestinal bacteria in the colon and absorbed. **Through the metabolic pathway, sc-FOS improves gastrointestinal (GI) condition such as relief from constipation, formation of preferable intestinal microflora and intestinal immunomodulation those are known as prebiotics' function. Besides improvement of GI condition, dietary sc-FOS influences on calcium and magnesium absorption in the colon. A major mineral absorption site is the small intestine, but the colon also works as a Ca and Mg absorption site with an aid of SCFAs made from sc-FOS.**

ＣＳＣＲＣＳＣＲ

FOS
Increases SCFAs and Friendly Bacteria

In the *Journal of Nutrition* 01-AUG-2005; 135(8): 1896-902

K Whelan, et al., studied

"Fructooligosaccharides and fiber partially prevent the alterations in fecal microbiota and short-chain fatty acid

concentrations caused by standard enteral formula in healthy humans."

Abstract:

The intestinal microbiota are important during enteral tube feeding because they exert colonization resistance and produce SCFAs. However, the effect of the enteral formula composition on major bacterial groups of the microbiota has not been clearly defined. The aim of this study was to investigate the effect of enteral formulas with and without prebiotic fructooligosaccharides (FOS) and fiber on the fecal microbiota and SCFAs. **This study demonstrates that standard enteral formula leads to adverse alterations to the fecal microbiota and SCFA concentrations in healthy subjects, and these alterations are partially prevented by fortification of the formula with FOS and fiber.**

ઉ૦ઉ૦

Oligoosaccharides
Increases calcium absorption and increases bone mineral density

In the *Journal of Nutrition* 01-FEB-2004; 134(2): 399-402

TA Zafar, et al., studied...

"Nondigestible oligosaccharides increase calcium absorption and suppress bone resorption in ovariecto-mized rats."

and found that...

Calcium absorption, femoral calcium content, BMD, and bone balance (V(bal)) were significantly increased (P < 0.05) by NDO, whereas the bone resorption rate relative to the bone formation rate was significantly depressed by NDO. We conclude that feeding NDO [Nondigestible oligosaccharides] **at**

5.5 g/100 g for 21 d has a positive effect on calcium absorption and retention in ovariectomized rats.

ME COMMENTS:

Loss of bone density actually starts before menopause. This study, with regards to surgically induced menopause, points out that FOS may be the treatment of choice instead of Fosamax® and its family of drugs. Fosamax® does not build new bone, it slows down the absorption of old bone. It is similar to putting a new coat of paint on a car that is rusted out.

ଔଋଔଋ

FOS

Increases cells lining intestinal wall

In the journal *Poultry Science* 01-JUN-2003; 82(6): 1030-6

ZR Xu, et al., studied...

"Effects of dietary fructooligosaccharide on digestive enzyme activities, intestinal microflora and morphology of male broilers."

Abstract:

Two hundred forty male Avian Farms broiler chicks, 1 day of age, were randomly allocated to four treatments, each of which had five pens of 12 chicks per pen. The chicks were used to investigate the effects of fructooligosaccharide (FOS) on digestive enzyme activities and intestinal microflora and morphology...

and found that...

addition of 4.0 g/kg FOS significantly increased ileal villus height, jejunal and ileal microvillus height, and villus-height-to-crypt-depth ratios at the jejunum and ileum and decreased crypt depth at the jejunum and ileum. However, addition of 8.0 g/kg FOS had no significant effect on growth

performance, digestive enzyme activities, intestinal microflora, or morphology.

ME COMMENTS:

By increasing the quantity of cells that line the intestines you lower the probability of pathogenic bacteria entering the blood stream.

ꟹꟹꟹꟹ

FOS, GOS & INFANT FORMULA

Stimulates the intestinal flora in bottle fed babies to simulate that of breastfed infants

In the *Journal of Clinical Gastroenterology* 01-JUL-2004; 38(6 Suppl): S76-9

G. Boehm, et al., studied...

"Prebiotics in infant formulas."

Abstract:

BACKGROUND: The intestinal flora of breast-fed infants is an important physiologic factor in the function of the gut and in the development of the immune system. The current research is part of a group of studies performed to answer the question whether a bovine milk formula supplemented with a prebiotic mixture from galactooligosaccharides and fructooligosaccharides can stimulate an intestinal flora similar to that of breast-fed infants...

...CONCLUSION: **The data obtained indicate that the prebiotic mixture under study is able to stimulate the development of a microbial flora similar to that of breast-fed infants.**

ME COMMENTS:

They don't seem to get it!!! It seems like they are more interested in adding substances to infant formula rather than encouraging breastfeeding. However, the scientists finally realized that breastfed babies have different bacteria in their intestine. This may be the reason why breastfed babies have fewer infections than bottle fed babies. (See Chapter on HMOs.)

ঌ৫ঌ৫

FOS

Increases the absorption of iron, magnesium and calcium

In the *Journal of Nutritional Science and Vitaminology* (Tokyo) (1995 Jun) 41(3):281-91

A. Ohta, et. al., studied...

"Effects of fructooligosaccharides on the absorption of iron, calcium and magnesium in iron-deficient anemic rats."

We investigated the effects of fructooligosaccharides (FO)-feeding on the absorption of iron (Fe), calcium (Ca) and magnesium (Mg) and on the biochemical parameters in Fe-deficient anemic rats. Fe-deficient anemic rats were made by feeding an Fe-deficient diet for 3 weeks. Then these Fe-deficient rats were fed an experimental diet that contained one of two levels of Fe (15 or 30 mg/kg diet), in the form of ferric pyrophosphate, and one of two levels of FO (0 or 50 g/kg diet) for 2 weeks. After the rats were fed these experimental diets, FO-feeding increased the hematocrit ratio, the concentration of hemoglobin and the hemoglobin regeneration efficiency during the first week. Also, the apparent absorption of Fe was increased by FO- feeding. The levels of Fe in the diet did not affect the absorption of Ca and Mg. However, FO-feeding increased the absorption of Ca and Mg. FO-feeding lowered the pH and raised the solubility of Fe, Ca and Mg in the cecal contents, suggesting that those increasing effects of FO-feeding on absorption of these minerals is correlated with fermentation of FO in the large intestine, namely, the cecum and colon. **We concluded that FO-feeding improved recovery from anemia and increased the absorption of Fe, Ca and Mg in Fe-deficient anemic rats.**

ME COMMENTS:

A truly incredible study with possible ramifications for the treatment of iron deficiency anemia in humans. In addition to iron supplementation, we should also be prescribing prebiotics like FOS.

ଔଔ

GOS

A treatment for constipation

In the journal *Annals of Nutrition & Metabolism* 1998;42:319-327

Ulla Teuria, et al., studied...

"Galactooligosaccharides Relieve Constipation in Elderly People"

Abstract

The aim of the study was to investigate whether galactooligosaccharides (GOS) relieve constipation in elderly people. The final study population consisted of 14 female subjects, mean age 79.6 (69-87) years, who suffered from constipation. The study was a double-blind two-period cross-over study. Both study periods lasted 2 weeks. The subjects ingested either 2 control yoghurts or 2 GOS-containing yoghurts daily. The yoghurts were otherwise similar, but the daily dose of GOS (Elix'or, BWP, Holland) from the GOS yoghurt was 9 g. **The regular use of laxatives was stopped during the study periods** and laxatives were used only when necessary. All the subjects reported the function of their intestines daily in a questionnaire. The defecation frequency per week (mean, range) was higher during the GOS period (7.1, 3-15) than during the control period (5.9, 1-14). GOS had no statistically significant effect on the use of laxatives, the consistency of feces or the ease of defecation, although GOS seemed to make defecation easier ($p = 0.07$). The adverse gastrointestinal symptoms were similar during both the control and the GOS periods. **GOS seem to relieve**

constipation in most elderly people but the responses differ individually.

ME COMMENTS:

I have found that FOS demonstrates a similar effect and is an excellent treatment for constipation in the entire population, including seniors.

ଔଓଔଓ

FOS

A treatment for diarrhea caused by Clostridium difficile

In the journal *Clinical Gastroenterology and Hepatology*, 01-MAY-2005; 3(5): 442-8

S. Lewis, et al., studied...

"Effect of the prebiotic oligofructose on relapse of Clostridium difficile-associated diarrhea: a randomized, controlled study."

Abstract:

BACKGROUND & AIMS: Ten percent to 20% of patients relapse after successful treatment of their Clostridium difficile -associated diarrhea. We set out to determine if the prebiotic oligofructose could alter the fecal bacterial flora and, in addition to antibiotic treatment, reduce the rate of relapse from Clostridium difficile infection. METHODS: Consecutive inpatients with Clostridium difficile - associated diarrhea were randomly allocated to receive oligofructose or placebo for 30 days in addition to specific antibiotic treatment. Patients were followed up for an additional 30 days. The main end point was the development of further diarrhea. Stools were collected for bacterial culture and Clostridium difficile toxin measurement...

...CONCLUSIONS: Fecal cultures confirmed the prebiotic effect of oligofructose (FOS). Patients taking oligofructose (FOS) were less likely to develop further diarrhea than those taking the placebo.

ME COMMENTS:

Clostridium difficile is a spore-forming, gram-positive bacillus that produces exotoxins that are pathogenic to humans. ***Clostridium difficile-disease (CDAD) ranges in severity from mild diarrhea to fulminant colitis and death. Antibiotic use is the primary risk factor*** *for development of CDAD because it disrupts normal bowel flora and promotes Clostridium difficile overgrowth. Clostridium difficile typically has affected older or severely ill patients who are hospital inpatients or residents of long term care facilities. Recently, however, both the frequency and severity of health care associated CDAD has increased. The CDC has received an increased number of reports of healthy individuals of all ages infected with Clostridium difficile.*

Clostridium difficile is becoming a serious problem, it's most serious side effect is diarrhea. The above study points out that another natural treatment (FOS) can help.

ଓଃଓଃ

MOS

Lowers pathogenic bacteria increases friendly bacteria

In *The American Society for Nutritional Sciences Journal of Nutrition* 2002,132:980-989

Kelly S. Swanson, et al., studied...

"Supplemental Fructooligosaccharides and Mannanoligosaccharides Influence Immune Function, Ileal and Total Tract Nutrient Digestibilities, Microbial Populations and Concentrations of Protein Catabolites in the Large Bowel of Dogs"

and found...

...Dogs supplemented with MOS had lower fecal total aerobes [pathogenic bacteria] and tended to have greater lactobacillus [friendly bacteria] populations...

ME COMMENTS:

Possibly by destroying their cell walls, MOS lowers the total count of pathogenic bacteria.

ઉ૩ઉ૩

MOS
A possible replacement for antibiotics in cows

In the journal of the American Dairy Science Association, Journal of Dairy Science 2003 86:4064-4069 .

A. J. Heinrichs, et al. studied...

"Effects of Mannan Oligosaccharide or Antibiotics in Neonatal Diets on Health and Growth of Dairy Calves"

and found...

Seventy-two Holstein calves were used to study the effect of feeding antibiotics or mannan oligosaccharides (MOS) in milk replacer... Addition of MOS or antibiotics increased the probability of normal scores for fecal fluidity, scours severity, and fecal consistency as compared to control calves during the course of the study... The results suggest that antibiotics in milk replacers can be replaced with compounds such as mannan oligosaccharides to obtain similar calf performance.

ME COMMENTS:

I believe these findings may also be applicable to humans.

ઉ૩ઉ૩

MOS
Alternative to antibiotics in pigs

In the Journal of Animal Science, 2005; 83(11):2637-44

DW, Rozeboom, et al., studied...

"Effects of mannan oligosaccharide and an antimicrobial product in nursery diets on performance of pigs reared on three different farms."

...The results of this study suggest that MOS may be an alternative to tylosin and sulfa-methazine [antibiotics] as a growth promotant in nursery diets.

ME COMMENTS:

One mode of action for mannanoligosaccharides involves interference with colonization of intestinal pathogens. Bacteria have lecithins (proteins or glycoproteins) on the cell surface that recognize specific sugars and allow the cell to attach to that sugar. These sugars can be found on the epithelial cell surface. Binding of Salmonella, Escherichia coli and Vibrio cholera has been shown to be mediated by a mannose-specific lecithin-like substance on the bacterial cell surface.

These studies on MOS have all been conducted on animals but the results most likely will be applicable to humans i.e. that MOS causes destruction of pathogenic bacteria by adhering to the cell wall and in the process destroying the bacteria.

OLIGOOSACCHARIDES
All have different characteristics

In the *Journal Applied Microbiology.* 2001 Nov;91(5):878-87.

CE Rycroft, et al., studied...

"A comparative in vitro evaluation of the fermentation properties of prebiotic oligosaccharides."

and found that...

...All prebiotics increased the numbers of bifidobacteria and most decreased clostridia. Xylooligosaccharides and lactulose produced the highest increases in numbers of bifidobacteria whilst fructooligosaccharides produced the highest populations of lactobacilli. Galactooligosaccharides (GOS) resulted in the largest decreases in numbers of clostridia.

ME COMMENTS:

We are seeing just the beginning of modern science realizing the importance and function of the different oligosaccharides. All oligosaccharides increase the number of both friendly bacteria and SCFAs. Further study will reveal their other beneficial attributes.

ଔଓଔଓ

FOS
and calcium absorption

In the *American Journal of Clinical Nutrition*, Vol. 69, No. 3, 544-548, March 1999

Ellen GHM van den Heuvel, et al., studied...

__**"Oligofructose stimulates calcium absorption in adolescents"**

and found...

Background: In rats, nondigestible oligosaccharides stimulate calcium absorption. Recently, this effect was also found in human subjects.

Objective: The objective of the study was to investigate whether consumption of 15 g oligofructose/d stimulates calcium absorption in male adolescents.

Conclusion: Fifteen grams of oligofructose per day stimulates fractional calcium absorption in male adolescents.

ME COMMENTS:

This scientific study shows that FOS not only stimulates calcium absorption in animals, but also in humans.

ଓଓ ଓଓ

FOS
and calcium absorption

In the *American Journal of Clinical Nutrition,* Vol. 82, No. 2, 471-476, August 2005

Steven A Abrams, et al., studied...

"A combination of prebiotic short- and long-chain inulin-type fructans enhances calcium absorption and bone mineralization in young adolescents"

and found...

...Conclusion: Daily consumption of a combination of prebiotic short- and long-chain inulin-type fructans significantly increases calcium absorption and enhances bone mineralization during pubertal growth. Effects of dietary factors on calcium absorption may be modulated by genetic factors, including specific vitamin D receptor gene polymorphisms.

ME COMMENTS:

This more recent scientific study confirms that FOS not only stimulates calcium absorption in animals, but also in humans.

ଔଔ

OLIGOSACCHARIDES and PROBIOTICS
Lowering cholesterol levels

In the *Journal of Applied Microbiology.* 2005; 98(5):1115-26

MT Liong, et al., studied...

"Optimization of cholesterol removal, growth and fermentation patterns of Lactobacillus acidophilus ATCC 4962 in the presence of mannitol, fructooligosaccharide and inulin: a response surface methodology approach."

and found...

CONCLUSIONS: Optimum cholesterol removal was obtained from the fermentation of L. acidophilus ATCC 4962 in the presence of mannitol, FOS and inulin. Cholesterol removal and the production of SCFA appeared to be growth associated and highly influenced by the prebiotics...

...The results provide better understanding on the interactions between probiotic and prebiotics for the removal of cholesterol.

ME COMMENTS:

This study shows that in order to lower cholesterol it is important to use Probiotics with your Prebiotics.

ଔଔ

HUMAN MILK OLIGOSACCHARIDES HMOs

> *"Breasts are more skillful at compounding a feeding mixture than the hemispheres of the most learned professor's brain."*
>
> *Oliver Wendell Holmes, M.D.*

For over 30 years, the cornerstone of my practice, Homefirst® Health Services, has been physician attended homebirth and promotion and encouragement of breastfeeding. I have been privileged to develop a practice of thousands of families who have had babies at home and have nursed their children for over two years. Since 1973 the physicians at Homefirst® Health Services have treated relatively few cases of ear infection, throat infection, allergy, eczema, etc. as compared to rates of these illnesses in a bottle fed population. One study found that the average physician sees one ear infection out of every five visits. We see one ear infection out of approximately 50 visits. The wisdom as to the benefits of breastfeeding most probably does not come to our patients from scientific articles. To these mothers, many of them LaLeche members and leaders, it is innately obvious that human breastmilk is for humans and cows milk is for cows.

The discovery of human milk oligosaccharides (HMOs), [this is like Columbus discovering America, as if it was never there] now gives scientific veracity to explaining why breastfed children are so healthy. In an outstanding editorial by Dr. Magdalana Araya, MD, PhD, in the September 2004 issue of the *Journal of Pediatrics* the concept of HMOs as a preventive measure is explored as to why breastfed children have far fewer illnesses than bottle fed children.

HMOs

Cow's milk is a poor carrier of bio-active fiber-fermenting probiotics because, in sharp contrast to breastmilk, it contains virtually no oligosaccharides (only elephant's milk contains as many oligosaccharides as human milk). The complex HMOs in human milk, protect breastfed infants against infection and inflammation. Breastmilk has over 130 different HMOs. Each is now believed to have a unique role in maintaining infant and newborn health. Sad to say, this natural resource is being wasted by feeding cow's milk, disguised as "formula", to human infants.

The breastfeeding rates in this country are dismally low. Less than 10% of newborns are being breastfed at 6 months. Maybe as doctors read in the current scientific journals about the "miraculous" endogenous prebiotics (HMOs), they will begin to insist on breastfeeding. I find it interesting that if a patient refuses to vaccinate their child, 30% of doctors say they will not care for them. Maybe medical professionals should put the same energy into the most important aspect of newborn nutrition, breastfeeding. Maybe they should refuse to see patients who do not follow the standards of the American Academy of Pediatrics, "exclusive breastfeeding until the infant is approximately six months of age, with timely introduction of complementary foods and continued breastfeeding to a year, or longer if desired."

The following scientific studies document the evidence based approach to understand the importance of HMOs.

ଔଓଔଓ

Oligosaccharides in Elephant Milk

In the *British Journal Nutrition* 1999 Nov;82(5):391-9.

C. Kunz, et al studied

"Lactose-derived oligosaccharides in the milk of elephants: comparison with human milk."

Human milk is commonly considered to be unique when compared with the milk of other species with regard to its high content of complex fucosylated and sialylated lactose-derived oligosaccharides [HMOs]....

...Elephant and human milks have high levels and unique patterns of oligosaccharides which may reflect the relative importance of these components in neonatal host defence, in endothelial leucocyte interactions or in brain development.

ଔଓଔଓ

HMOs: only the breast

In the *Journal of Paediatrics and Child Health.* 1997 Aug;33(4):281-6.

P. McVeagh, et al. studied...

"Human milk oligosaccharides: only the breast."

New Children's Hospital, Westmead, Australia.

Over 100 years ago it was first deduced that a major component of human milk must be an unidentified carbohydrate that was not found in cows milk. At first this was thought to be a form of lactose and was called gynolactose. We now know that this was not a single carbohydrate but a complex mixture of approximately 130 different oligosaccharides. Although small amounts of a few oligosaccharides have been found in the milk of other mammals, this rich diversity of sugars is unique to human milk. The oligosaccharide content of human milk varies with the infant's gestation, the duration of lactation, diurnally and with the genetic makeup of the mother. Milk oligosaccharides have a number of functions that may protect the health of the breast fed infant. As they are not digested in the small intestine, they form the 'soluble' fibre of breast milk and their intact structure is available to act as competitive ligands protecting the breast-fed infant from pathogens. There is a growing list of pathogens for which a specific oligosaccharide ligand has been described in human milk. They are likely to form the model for future therapeutic and prophylactic anti-microbials. They provide substrates for bacteria in the infant colon and thereby contribute to the difference in faecal pH and faecal flora between breast and formula-fed infants. They may also be important as a source of sialic acid, essential for brain development.

ઉ૨ઉ૨

HMOs and infections

In *The Journal of Pediatrics* September 2004

Magdalena Araya, MD, PhD, studied

Excerpts from Editorial

"NOVEL OLIGOSACCHARIDES IN HUMAN MILK: UNDERSTANDING MECHANISMS MAY LEAD TO BETTER PREVENTION OF ENTERIC AND OTHER INFECTIONS"

...Human milk is known to contain significant amounts of over 130 lactose-derived oligosaccharides, whilst cows' milk contains only trace amounts... Some HMO are known to be potent inhibitors of bacterial adhesion to epithelial cells by acting as receptor analogues to mucosal adhesion molecules... From this, it can be postulated that HMO may contribute towards the lower incidence of gastrointestinal, respiratory and urinary infections seen in breast-fed infants compared with those who are formula-fed...

...Every year scientists find new substances which are unique to breastmilk and they try to add them to a variety of infant formulas instead of absolutely recommending breastfeeding. The protective, as well as, nutritive properties of breastmilk have been known for a long time. The emergence of interest in Probiotics has brought illumination to how the protective properties of breastmilk work.

...The newborn will first come in contact with bacteria from the birth canal and its surroundings. Factors such as microbial flora of the female genital tract, sanitary conditions, obstetric techniques, vaginal or Caesarean mode of delivery, geographical distribution of bacterial species and type of feeding all have an effect on the level and frequency of various species colonising the infant gut.

ঙঙঙঙ

HMOs and infectious diarrhea

In the journal *Seminars Pediatric Infectious Disease* - 01-OCT-2004; 15(4): 221-8

AL Morrow, et al., studied

"Human milk protection against infectious diarrhea: implications for prevention and clinical care."

Abstract:

Breastfeeding is the major strategy for prevention of morbidity and mortality resulting from diarrhea in the first few years of life. Health-system and community based interventions have been shown to increase the prevalence of breastfeeding and reduce the incidence of diarrhea and associated healthcare costs in infancy. The protective effect of breastfeeding is attributable to a complex of acquired and innate factors unique to human milk that have anti-infective, anti-inflammatory, and immunoregulatory functions, including secretory antibodies, oligosaccharides, glycoconjugates, lactoferrin, leukocytes, cytokines, and other agents. The American Academy of Pediatrics recommends exclusive breastfeeding until the infant is approximately 6 months of age, with timely introduction of complementary foods and continued breastfeeding to a year, or longer if desired. **The number of deaths of children that could be prevented worldwide each year if these breastfeeding recommendations were followed has been estimated to be more than 1 million.**

ME COMMENTS:

Why are the world health medical organizations not putting more energy into promoting breastfeeding? A simple answer - the only person who benefits from breastfeeding is the baby, not the bottom line profits or bank accounts of major pharmaceutical companies.

ও৪ও৪

HMOs and infectious diarrhea

In the *Journal of Nutrition* 01-MAY-2005; 135(5): 1304-7

AL Morrow, et al., studied...

"Human-milk glycans that inhibit pathogen binding protect breast-feeding infants against infectious diarrhea."

Abstract:

Breast-feeding is a highly effective strategy for preventing morbidity and mortality in infancy. The human-milk glycans, which include oligosaccharides in their free and conjugated forms, constitute a major and an innate immunologic mechanism by which human milk protects breast-fed infants against infections. The glycans found in human milk function as soluble receptors that inhibit pathogens from adhering to their target receptors on the mucosal surface of the host gastrointestinal tract. The alpha1,2-linked fucosylated glycans, which require the secretor gene for expression in human milk, are the dominant glycan structure found in the milk of secretor mothers, who constitute the majority (approximately 80%) of mothers worldwide. In vitro and in vivo binding studies have demonstrated that alpha1,2-linked fucosylated glycans inhibit binding by campylobacter, stable toxin of enterotoxigenic Escherichia coli, and major strains of caliciviruses to their target host cell receptors. Consistent with these findings, recently published epidemiologic data demonstrate that higher relative concentrations of alpha1,2-linked fucosylated glycans in human milk are associated with protection of breast-fed infants against diarrhea caused by campylobacter, caliciviruses, and stable toxin of enterotoxigenic E. coli, and moderate-to-severe diarrhea of all causes. These novel data open the potential for translational research to develop the human-milk glycans as a new class of antimicrobial agents that prevent infection by acting as pathogen anti-adhesion agents.

ଓଃଓଃ

HMOs and infectious diseases

In the *Annual Review of Nutrition* 01-JAN-2005; 25: 37-58

DS Newburg , et al., studied

"Human milk glycans protect infants against enteric pathogens."

Abstract:

Breastfed infants have lower morbidity and mortality due to diarrhea than those fed artificially. This had been attributed primarily to the secretory antibodies and prebiotic factors in human milk. Oligosaccharides are the third largest component of human milk. They were initially considered to be functionless by-products of glycoprotein and glycolipid synthesis during milk production. However, in the past few decades it has become apparent that the human milk oligosaccharides are composed of thousands of components, at least some of which protect against pathogens. Oligosaccharide protection against infectious agents may result in part from their prebiotic characteristics, but is thought to be primarily due to their inhibition of pathogen binding to host cell ligands. Most human milk oligosaccharides are fucosylated, and their production depends on enzymes encoded by the genes associated with expression of the Lewis blood group system. The expression of specific fucosylated oligosaccharides in milk thus varies in relation to maternal Lewis blood group type, and is significantly associated with the risk of infectious disease in breastfed infants. Specific fucosylated moieties of oligosaccharides and related glycoconjugates (glycans) are able to inhibit binding and disease by specific pathogens. This review presents the argument that specific glycans, especially the oligosaccharides, are the major constituent of an innate immune system of human milk whereby the mother protects her infant from enteric and other pathogens through breastfeeding. The large input of energy expended by the mother in the synthesis of milk oligosaccharides is consistent with the human reproductive strategy of large parental input into rearing relatively few offspring through a prolonged period of maturation. These protective glycans may prove useful as a basis for the development of novel prophylactic and therapeutic agents that inhibit diseases caused by mucosal pathogens.

ᏈᏡᏈᏡ

HMOs and infant diarrhea

In the *Journal of Pediatrics* Volume 145, Issue 3, Pages 297-303 (September 2004)

Guillermo M. Ruiz-Palacios, et al., studied

"Human milk oligosaccharides are associated with protection against diarrhea in breast-fed infants"

Objective: To determine the association between maternal milk levels of 2-linked fucosylated oligosaccharide and prevention of diarrhea as a result of Campylobacter, caliciviruses, and diarrhea of all causes in breast-fed infants.

Study design: Data and banked samples were analyzed from 93 breast-feeding mother-infant pairs who were prospectively studied during 1988-1991 from birth to 2 years with infant feeding and diarrhea data collected weekly; diarrhea was diagnosed by a study physician. Milk samples obtained 1 to 5 weeks postpartum were analyzed for oligosaccharide content. Data were analyzed by Poisson regression.

Conclusion: This study provides novel evidence suggesting that human milk oligosaccharides are clinically relevant to protection against infant diarrhea.

ᏈᏡᏈᏡ

HMOs and infant diarrhea

In the *Journal of Pediatrics*, Volume 145, Issue 3, Pages 297-303 (September 2004)

Dr. Ardythe L. Morrow, et al., studied

"Human milk oligosaccharides are associated with protection against diarrhea in breastfed infants"

Objective: To determine the association between maternal milk levels of 2-linked fucosylated oligosaccharide and prevention of diarrhea as a result of Campylobacter, caliciviruses, and diarrhea of all causes in breast-fed infants.

Study design: Data and banked samples were analyzed from 93 breast-feeding mother-infant pairs who were prospectively studied during 1988-1991 from birth to 2 years with infant feeding and diarrhea data collected weekly; diarrhea was diagnosed by a study physician. Milk samples obtained 1 to 5 weeks postpartum were analyzed for oligosaccharide content. Data were analyzed by Poisson regression.

Conclusion: This study provides novel evidence suggesting that human milk oligosaccharides are clinically relevant to protection against infant diarrhea.

ME COMMENTS:

While I agree with the conclusion, unfortunately Dr. Morrow has it backwards. HMOs don't protect the breastfeeding babies from diarrhea, the lack of HMOs in cow's milk formula cause it!

Human Milk Probiotics

In the *Journal of Pediatrics.* 01-DEC-2003; 143(6): 754-8

R. Martín, et. al., studied...

"Human milk is a source of lactic acid bacteria for the infant gut."

Abstract:

OBJECTIVES: To investigate whether human breast milk contains potentially probiotic lactic acid bacteria, and therefore, whether it can be considered a synbiotic food. Study design Lactic acid bacteria were isolated from milk, mammary areola, and breast skin of eight healthy mothers and oral swabs and feces of their respective breast-fed infants. Some isolates (178 from each mother and newborn pair) were randomly selected and submitted to randomly amplified polymorphic DNA (RAPD) polymerase chain reaction analysis, and those that displayed identical RAPD patterns were identified by 16S rDNA sequencing.

RESULTS: Within each mother and newborn pair, some rod-shaped lactic acid bacteria isolated from mammary areola, breast milk, and infant oral swabs and feces displayed identical RAPD profiles. All of them, independently from the mother and child pair, were identified as Lactobacillus gasseri. Similarly, among coccoid lactic acid bacteria from these different sources, some shared an identical RAPD pattern and were identified as Enterococcus faecium. In contrast, none of the lactic acid bacteria isolated from breast skin shared RAPD profiles with lactic acid bacteria of the other sources.

CONCLUSIONS: Breast-feeding can be a significant source of lactic acid bacteria to the infant gut. Lactic acid bacteria present in milk may have an endogenous origin and may not be the result of contamination from the surrounding breast skin.

ଔଔ

ME COMMENTS ON HMOs:

Cow's milk for cows, human's milk for humans. Many doctors still believe that God made a mistake by not putting Enfamil® into womens' breasts. The high rate of Cesarean Sections also robs newborns of the opportunity to colonize healthy bacteria, as the baby does not pass through the birth canal. There is also an increased body of evidence which suggests that HMOs (human milk oligosaccharides) present in breast milk may act as decoys for bacterial toxins and disease causing bacteria in infants. Some investigators have found that these complex sugars found in breastmilk, act as scavengers - collecting, removing and neutralizing disease causing bacteria toxins.

SCFA
(Short Chain Fatty Acids)

A majority of the benefits of friendly bacteria are the production of SCFAs. Remember that humans cannot break down prebiotics, i.e. FOS, MOS, etc. However, the fermentation of the oligosaccharides by friendly bacteria results in the SCFAs which can be broken down by humans and used as an energy source. The most common of the SCFAs are acetic acid, proprionic acid, buteryic acid, and to a lesser extent lactic acid. Antibiotics can impair the process of fermentation in the colon thereby lowering the production of SCFAs. Antibiotics not only kill off pathogenic bacteria, they kill off friendly bacteria. This is the reason why you cannot take probiotics together with antibiotics; you must take them at least two hours apart. Diarrhea also reduces the amount of SCFAs as it shortens the amount of time the food is in the large intestine thus reducing the amount of time available for fermentation.

Some of the scientific studies have pointed out the following benefits of SCFAs:

1. A source of energy for growing friendly bacteria
2. A source of energy for the epithelial cells that line the colon
3. Butyric acid has been shown to stimulate growth of epithelial cells that line the colon
4. Butyric acid has been shown to slow the grown of cancer cells in the intestine
5. Butyric acid may trigger apoptosis of cancer cells
6. Butyric acid has been shown to facilitate cell repair
7. Butyric acid has been shown to protect against colon and rectal cancer

8. SCFAs prevent overgrowth of pathogenic bacteria by making the environment of the large intestine more acidic
9. SCFAs may play a role in lowering blood sugar and blood cholesterol levels

The following scientific studies document the evidence based approach to understanding the benefits of SCFAs.

☙❧☙❧

SCFAs and Cholesterol

In the *Journal of Nutrition*. 1999;129:942-948.

Hiroshi Hara1, et al., studied...

"Short-Chain Fatty Acids Suppress Cholesterol Synthesis in Rat Liver and Intestine"

We previously showed that plasma cholesterol levels decreased following ingestion of a short-chain fatty acid (SCFA) mixture composed of sodium salts of acetic, propionic, and butyric acids simulating cecal fermentation products of sugar-beet fiber (SBF). In the present study, we investigated whether hepatic and small intestinal cholesterol synthesis is involved in the cholesterol-lowering effects of SCFA and SBF....

...These results show that a decrease in hepatic cholesterol synthesis rate mainly contributes to the lowering of plasma cholesterol in rats fed the SCFA mixture diet. Changes in portal SCFA and cholesterol concentrations support this conclusion. In SBF-fed rats, SCFA produced by cecal fermentation are possibly involved in lowering plasma cholesterol levels by negating the counteractive induction of hepatic cholesterol synthesis caused by an increase in bile acid excretion.

ME COMMENTS:

Another study to show that SCFAs lower cholesterol levels in rats and these results most probably carry over to humans. SCFAs are naturally produced by the endogenous as well exogenous friendly bacteria in the colon. They are also produced by probiotics and can be taken as a supplement. Prebiotics such as FOS will feed both types of friendly bacteria and thus increase the production of SCFAs.

SCFAs and Colon Cancer

In the *Journal of Nutrition.* 132:1012-1017, 2002

Brian F. Hinnebusch, et al., studied...

"The Effects of Short-Chain Fatty Acids on Human Colon Cancer Cell Phenotype are Associated with Histone Hyperacetylation"

The short-chain fatty acid (SCFA) butyrate is produced via anaerobic bacterial fermentation within the colon and is thought to be protective in regard to colon carcinogenesis. Although butyrate (C4) is considered the most potent of the SCFA, a variety of other SCFA also exist in the colonic lumen. Butyrate is thought to exert its cellular effects through the induction of histone hyperacetylation. We sought to determine the effects of a variety of the SCFA on colon carcinoma cell growth, differentiation and apoptosis. HT-29 or HCT-116 (wild-type and p21-deleted) cells were treated with physiologically relevant concentrations of various SCFA, and histone acetylation state was assayed by acid-urea-triton-X gel electrophoresis and immunoblotting. Growth and apoptotic effects were studied by flow cytometry, and differentiation effects were assessed using transient transfections and Northern blotting. Propionate (C3) and valerate (C5) caused growth arrest and differentiation in human colon carcinoma cells. The magnitude of their effects was associated with a lesser degree of histone hyperacetylation compared with butyrate. Acetate (C2) and caproate (C6), in contrast, did not cause histone hyperacetylation and also had no appreciable effects on cell growth or differentiation. SCFA-induced transactivation of the differentiation marker gene, intestinal alkaline phosphatase (IAP), was blocked by histone deacetylase (HDAC), further supporting the critical link between SCFA and histones. Butyrate also significantly increased apoptosis, whereas the other SCFA studied did not. The growth arrest induced by the SCFA was characterized by an increase in the expression of the p21 cell-cycle inhibitor and down-regulation of cyclin B1 (CB1). In p21-deleted HCT-116 colon cancer cells, the

SCFA did not alter the rate of proliferation. These data suggest that the antiproliferative, apoptotic and differentiating properties of the various SCFA are linked to the degree of induced histone hyper-acetylation. Furthermore, SCFA-mediated growth arrest in colon carcinoma cells requires the p21 gene....

...In conclusion, we have determined the relative effects of a variety of SCFA on histone acetylation, cellular growth arrest, differentiation and apoptosis in colon carcinoma cells. Our results clearly point to the importance of the histone-modifying effects of SCFA. Because different types of dietary fiber produce varying amounts of the specific SCFA, it is likely that the exact composition of fiber within the colonic lumen may determine its cellular effects, including its possible beneficial role in the prevention and/or treatment of colon cancer.

ME COMMENTS:

An interesting area of scientific research looking at the role of SCFAs in the prevention of colon cancer.

SCFAs and Colon Cancer

In the journal *Biochemical Pharmacology* 1997 May 9;53(9):1357-68.

JA McBain, et al. studied...

"Apoptotic death in adenocarcinoma cell lines induced by butyrate and other histone deacetylase inhibitors."

n-Butyrate inhibits the growth of colon cancer cell lines....

...Thus, applications of butyrate for cytoreduction therapy will benefit from pharmacodynamic assessment of histone acetylation, but will require additional work to predict susceptibility to butyrate-induced death.

ME COMMENTS:

n-Butyrate is a small chain fatty acid (SCFA) produced by the friendly bacteria in our intestine, as well as available as a natural pharmaceutical. This study points out one of the many benefits of the SCFAs.

ങരങര

SCFAs and Colon Cancer

In the *Chinese Journal of Digestive Diseases*, 01-JAN-2004; 5(3): 115-7

H FU, et. al., studied...

"Effect of short-chain fatty acids on the proliferation and differentiation of the human colonic adenocarcinoma cell line Caco-2."

Abstract:

OBJECTIVE: Short-chain fatty acids (SCFA) in the colon may maintain colonocyte differentiation and oppose carcinogenesis. The purpose of this study was to investigate the effects of three SCFA, butyrate, propionate and acetate, on the differentiation, proliferation, and matrix interactions of the Caco-2 human colonic adenocarcinoma cell line.

METHODS: Differentiation was assessed by brush border enzyme expression and the doubling time (proliferation) was calculated directly from serial cell counts and by the logarithmic transformation method. Cell motility (migration) was quantitated by the expansion of a confluent Caco-2 monolayer (after release from a constraining fence) across bacteriologic plastic dishes precoated with saturating concentrations of type I collagen. Results were expressed as mean +/- SE and were analyzed by ANOVA and Bonferroni's modified t-test.

RESULTS: All three SCFA studied altered the Caco-2 phenotype. Treatment with 10 mmol SCFA significantly prolonged the cell doubling time, promoted brush border enzyme expression (cathepsin C), and inhibited the motility of the Caco-2 cells.

CONCLUSIONS: Butyrate, propionate and acetate inhibited the proliferation and motility of a well-differentiated human colonic cancer cell line while promoting the expression of the differentiation marker, cathepsin C. **Thus the SCFA produced by bacterial fermentation of dietary fiber may exert a protective effect against the development of colon cancer.**

ME COMMENTS:

Another study showing that SCFAs may be one of the answers to colon cancer prevention.

☙❧☙❧

SCFAs and Coccidiosis

In the journal *Poultry Science*, 01-SEP-2005; 84(9): 1418-22

S. Leeson, et al., studied...

"Effect of butyric acid on the performance and carcass yield of broiler chickens."

Abstract:

Short-chain fatty acids such as butyrate are considered potential alternatives to antibiotic growth promoters. The efficacy of butyric acid on performance and carcass characteristics of broiler chickens was tested in two studies. The effect of dietary butyrate on the ability to withstand coccidial oocyte challenge also was investigated. In experiment 1, male broiler chickens were fed diets supplemented with 0 or 11 ppm virginiamycin or 0.2 or 0.4% butyric acid (as mono-, di-, and triglyceride). In experiment 2, broilers were fed bacitracin methylene disalicylate or 0.1 or 0.2% butyric acid. In another trial, birds vaccinated against coccidiosis were challenged with oocytes at 21 d and examined 6 d later. In experiment 1, diet treatments had no effect on body weight gain. Feed intake of the birds fed 0.4% butyric acid was decreased ($P < 0.01$) compared with birds fed the nonmedicated diet during the starter period, whereas birds fed 0.2% butyric acid had similar feed intake to the control birds. In experiment 2, diet treatments did not affect the performance of broiler chicks while carcass weight and breast meat yield increased ($P < 0.01$) in birds fed 0.2% butyric acid. With oocyte challenge, birds that had received butyric acid before challenge showed higher growth rate following the challenge compared with birds that received nonmedicated feed. Bacitracin decreased ($P < 0.05\%$) duodenal villi crypt depth, whereas villus length was similar in birds fed butyric acid or the nonmedicated control diet. **These results show that 0.2% butyric acid can help to maintain the performance and carcass quality of broilers, especially in vaccinated birds challenged with coccidiosis.**

ઉઙઉઙ

SCFAs and Epithelial Cell Growth in the Large Intestine

In the *Journal of Nutritional Science and Vitaminology*, (Tokyo) 01-JUN-2005; 51(3): 156-60

A. Inagaki, et al., studied...

"Dose-dependent stimulatory and inhibitory effects of luminal and serosal n-butyric acid on epithelial cell proliferation of pig distal colonic mucosa."

Abstract:

Large bowel bacteria convert various carbohydrates into short-chain fatty acids (SCFA). SCFA stimulate epithelial cell proliferation of the large intestine in vivo and inhibit that of various cells in vitro. Supposing that too high concentration of SCFA on the serosal side is responsible for their inhibitory effect in vitro, we studied effects of luminal and serosal n-butyric acid (0, 0.1, 1, or 10 mmol/L, adjusted to neutral pH) on the epithelial cell proliferation rate of pig colonic mucosa in organ culture taking crypt cell production rate (CCPR) as the measure of proliferative activity. With 0 or 0.1 mmol/L n-butyric acid on the serosal side, luminal n-butyric acid increased CCPR at 1.0 mmol/L, and decreased CCPR at 10 mmol/L when compared to the luminal 0 mmol/L control. With 1.0 or 10 mmol/L serosal n-butyric acid, luminal n-butyric acid depressed CCPR dose-dependently. The above results indicated that n-butyric acid stimulated colonic epithelial cell proliferation at low concentration and inhibit it at high concentration with interaction effect to enhance the inhibitory action. **The stimulatory effect of a low dose of serosal n-butyric acid may be responsible for the distant trophic effect of SCFA.**

ME COMMENTS:

SCFAs increase cellular growth in the large intestine, thereby creating a buffer zone against unfriendly bacteria trying to enter the body.

Notes

MUSCLE & JOINT PAIN

Millions of American suffer from muscle and joint pain, from the weekend warriors to the severely arthritic. Billions of dollars are spent on drug pharmaceuticals such as: Vioxx®, Bextra®, Celebrex®, Mobid®, NSAIDS, aspirin, Tylenol®. The medications have side effects which include: fever, sneezing, chest congestion, cough, sore throat, swelling in the arms and legs, trouble sleeping, dizziness, lack of appetite, diarrhea, difficulty breathing, yellowing of the skin, eye problems, sluggishness, fatigue, unexplained weight gain, heart attacks, etc.

Today, there are over 9,500 lawsuits filed against Merck claiming that the drug Vioxx® caused heart disease. Natural substitutes like Cetyl Myristoleate, Collagen Type II, Glucosamine, MSM, and Boswellia are just some of the alternatives to the drug pharmaceuticals. There have been no known reported major side effects with any of these natural pharmaceuticals, THAT'S THE BIG ADVANTAGE!

Cetyl Myristoleate is derived from an environmentally friendly source, palmitic acid (a fatty acid in coconut and palm oils). Cetyl myristoleate is a powerful anti-inflammatory agent. Additionally, it acts as a highly effective lubricant in joints, muscles and other tissues, allowing them to move more smoothly. It is also an immune system modulator which can be effective against auto-immune conditions. All of these characteristics contribute to its ability to act as an analgesic by removing the source of pain (inflamed and irritated tissues) so that there is no pain.

Collagen Type II is a dietary supplement that supports skin, joint and connective tissue health. It is naturally rich in Hyaluronic Acid (HA) a Cartilage Matrix Glycoprotein (TMGP), powerful substances that help protect the cartilage from breakdown and promote cartilage synthesis.

Glucosamine is an amino sugar normally formed in the body from glucose. It is the starting point for the synthesis of glycosaminoglycans (GAGs), including Hyaluronic Acid, a main constituent of joint fluid. Glucosamine supplementation can help support the thick gelatinous nature of the joint fluid, as well as proper functioning of joints, spinal disc, and other connective tissue.

MSM (Methyl Sulfonyl Methane) Complex is a naturally occurring sulfur compound that has a vitamin like normalizing influence on body functions. It can regulate pro-inflammatory enzymes to reduce pain and swelling associated with connective tissue dysfunction

Boswellia is a naturally occurring resin of the Boswellia serrata tree which grows in the dry hills of India. Preparations made from a purified extract of this substance are used to reduce inflammation associated with osteoarthritis and rheumatoid arthritis. Unlike conventional NSAIDs, such as ibuprofen, boswellia has no known side effects and does not seem to cause stomach irritation. It also may be effective for back pain and certain chronic intestinal disorders.

Scientific studies have shown that these natural pharmaceuticals actually work. However, there is a simpler test. If the muscle and joint pain go away - they work. If the muscle and joint pain are not relieved - they do not work. In my experience, various combinations of these natural pharmaceuticals for muscle and joint pain will help 75-80% of persons. The other 20-25% will require prescription pharmaceuticals. There is no one answer for everyone. However, with natural pharmaceuticals we surely will be able to help people with mild muscle and joint pain and even some with more pronounced muscle and joint pain.

The following scientific studies document the evidence based approach to using natural pharmaceuticals for muscle and joint pain.

ઉઌઉઌ

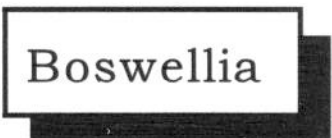

In the journal *Phytomedicine.* 2003; 10(1):3-7

N. Kimmatkar, et al., studied...

"Efficacy and tolerability of Boswellia serrata extract in treatment of osteoarthritis of knee--a randomized double blind placebo controlled trial."

Osteoarthritis is a common, chronic, progressive, skeletal, degenerative disorder, which commonly affects the knee joint. Boswellia serrata tree is commonly found in India. The therapeutic value of its gum (guggulu) has been known. It posses good anti-inflammatory, anti-arthritic and analgesic activity. A randomized double blind placebo controlled crossover study was conducted to assess the efficacy, safety and tolerability of Boswellia serrata Extract (BSE) in 30 patients of osteoarthritis of knee, 15 each receiving active drug or placebo for eight weeks. After the first intervention, washout was given and then the groups were crossed over to receive the opposite intervention for eight weeks. All patients receiving drug treatment reported decrease in knee pain, increased knee flexion and increased walking distance. The frequency of swelling in the knee joint was decreased. Radiologically there was no change. The observed differences between drug treated and placebo being statistically significant, are clinically relevant. BSE was well tolerated by the subjects except for minor gastrointestinal ADRs. **BSE is recommended in the patients of osteoarthritis of the knee with possible therapeutic use in other arthritis.**

ঙ৩ঙ৩

Boswellia

In the *Journal of Alternative and Complementary Medicine*, 2005; 11(2):323-31

AY Fan, et al., studied...

"Effects of an acetone extract of Boswellia carterii Birdw. (Burseraceae) gum resin on rats with persistent inflammation."

OBJECTIVE: Ruxiang, or Gummi olibanum, an herbal medicine derived from the gum resin of Boswellia carterii Birdw. (BC) of the family Burseraceae, has been used traditionally in China to alleviate pain and reduce inflammation. The present study is an investigation of the effects of a BC extract on persistent hyperalgesia and edema in rats with peripheral inflammation.

RESULTS: Compared to control, a dosage of 0.45 g/kg BC significantly lengthened PWL and reduced paw edema on day 5 post-CFA. At 0.90 g/kg, BC significantly lengthened PWL at 5 hours, 1 day, and 5 days, and reduced paw edema at 2 hours, 5 hours, 1 day, and 5 days. This dosage also significantly suppressed spinal Fos expression in the medial half of laminae I-II. At 1.80 g/kg, BC significantly lengthened PWL and reduced paw edema at all time points. No noticeable adverse effects were observed in animals given the lower dosages of BC, but adverse effects in some animals were observed at 1.80 g/kg per day. In the acute toxicity study, the maximal single dose of 2.50 g/kg produced no adverse effects in the treated rats during the 14 days of observation.

CONCLUSIONS: The data suggest that BC produces significant antihyperalgesia and anti-inflammation effects and that the antihyperalgesia may be mediated by suppressed inflammation-induced Fos expression in the spinal dorsal horn neurons.

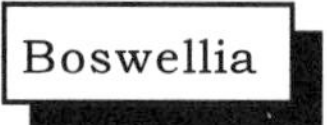

In the journal *DNA and Cell Biology*, 2005; 24(4):244-55

S. Roy, et al., studied...

"Human genome screen to identify the genetic basis of the anti-inflammatory effects of Boswellia in microvascular endothelial cells."

Inflammatory disorders represent a substantial health problem. Medicinal plants belonging to the Burseraceae family, including Boswellia, are especially known for their anti-inflammatory properties. The gum resin of Boswellia serrata contains boswellic acids, which inhibit leukotriene biosynthesis. A series of chronic inflammatory diseases are perpetuated by leukotrienes. Although Boswellia extract has proven to be anti-inflammatory in clinical trials, the underlying mechanisms remain to be characterized. TNF alpha represents one of the most widely recognized mediators of inflammation. One mechanism by which TNFalpha causes inflammation is by potently inducing the expression of adhesion molecules such as VCAM-1. We sought to test the genetic basis of the anti-inflammatory effects of BE (standardized Boswellia extract, 5-Loxin) in a system of TNF alpha-induced gene expression in human microvascular endothelial cells. We conducted the first whole genome screen for TNF alpha- inducible genes in human microvascular cells (HMEC). Acutely, TNF alpha induced 522 genes and downregulated 141 genes in nine out of nine pairwise comparisons. Of the 522 genes induced by TNF alpha in HMEC, 113 genes were clearly sensitive to BE treatment. Such genes directly related to inflammation, cell adhesion, and proteolysis. The robust BE-sensitive candidate genes were then subjected to further processing for the identification of BE-sensitive signaling pathways. The use of resources such as GenMAPP, KEGG, and gene ontology led to the recognition of the primary BE-sensitive TNF alpha-inducible pathways. BE prevented the TNF alpha-induced expression of matrix metalloproteinases. BE also prevented the inducible expression of mediators of apoptosis. Most strikingly, however, TNF alpha-inducible expression of VCAM-1 and ICAM-1 were observed to be sensitive to BE. Realtime PCR studies showed that while TNF alpha potently induced VCAM-1 gene expression, BE completely prevented it. **This result confirmed our microarray findings and built a compelling case for the anti-inflammatory property of BE.** In an in vivo model of carrageenan-induced rat paw inflammation, we observed a significant anti-inflammatory property of BE consistent with our in vitro findings. These findings warrant further research aimed at identifying the signaling mechanisms by which BE exerts its anti-inflammatory effects.

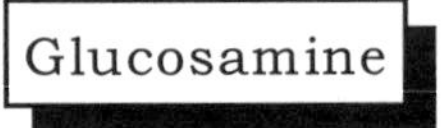

In the journal *Drugs & Aging.* 2003; 20(14):1041-60

AJ Matheson, et al., studied...

"Glucosamine: a review of its use in the management of osteoarthritis."

Glucosamine occurs naturally in all human tissues. It stimulates the synthesis of glycosaminoglycan, proteoglycan and hyaluronic acid, although the precise mechanism of action remains to be established. Formulated as glucosamine sulphate (Dona) and various others), glucosamine has been evaluated for its efficacy in relieving the symptoms of osteoarthritis and its disease-modifying potential. In two large randomised, double-blind, multicentre studies in patients with osteoarthritis, oral or intramuscular glucosamine for 4-6 weeks was associated with a greater decrease in symptom severity...

...Statistically significant differences favouring glucosamine were noted in the per- protocol and intention-to-treat analyses for the primary endpoints for both joint structural changes and symptom modification. Glucosamine has a tolerability profile similar to that of placebo and is better tolerated than ibuprofen or piroxicam. In particular, glucosamine recipients had a markedly lower incidence of gastrointestinal disturbances than those receiving ibuprofen. Other adverse events reported in both glucosamine and ibuprofen recipients were pruritus or skin reactions, flushing and fatigue. In general, a lower incidence of withdrawal from clinical trials was reported for glucosamine recipients than either ibuprofen or piroxicam recipients.

CONCLUSION: In short-term clinical trials, glucosamine provided effective symptomatic relief for patients with osteoarthritis of the knee. In addition, glucosamine has shown promising results in modifying the progression of arthritis over a 3-year period. Glucosamine may therefore prove to be a useful treatment option for osteoarthritis.

ଔଓଔଓ

Cetyl Myristoleate

In the *Journal of Rheumatology.* 01-APR-2004; 31(4): 767-74

WJ Kraemer, et.al., studied...

"Effect of a cetylated fatty acid topical cream on functional mobility and quality of life of patients with osteoarthritis."

Abstract:

OBJECTIVE: To examine the effect of a topical cream consisting of cetylated fatty acids on functional performance in patients diagnosed with osteoarthritis (OA) of one or both knees...

...RESULTS: For stair climbing ability and the up-and-go test, significant decreases in time were observed at T2 and T3 compared to T1 in the CFA group only. These differences were significant between groups. Supine ROM of the knees increased at T2 and T3 in CFA group, whereas no difference was observed in the placebo group. For the medial step-down test, significant improvement was observed at T2 and T3 compared to T1 in CFA group. For the unilateral anterior reach, significant improvement was observed for both legs in CFA group and in only the left leg in the placebo group. However, the improvements observed in CFA group were significantly greater than placebo group for both legs.

CONCLUSION: Use of a CFA topical cream is an effective treatment for improving knee ROM, ability to ascend/descend stairs, ability to rise from sitting, walk and sit down, and unilateral balance.

ଔଓଔଓ

Cetyl Myristoleate

In the *Journal of Rheumatology*. 2002 Aug;29(8):1708-12.

R. Hesslink, Jr., et al. studied...

"Cetylated Fatty Acids Improve Knee Function in Patients with Osteoarthritis"

OBJECTIVE: To determine the benefit of cetylated fatty acids (CFA) on knee range of motion and function in patients with osteoarthritis (OA).

METHODS: Sixty-four patients with chronic knee OA were evaluated at baseline and at 30 and 68 days after consuming either placebo (vegetable oil; n = 31) or CFA (Celadrin; n = 33). Evaluations included physician assessment, knee range of motion with goniometry, and the Lequesne Algofunctional Index (LAI)...

...CONCLUSION: Compared to placebo, CFA provides an improvement in knee range of motion and overall function in patients with OA of the knee. CFA may be an alternative to the use of nonsteroidal anti-inflammatory drugs for the treatment of OA.

ଔଓଔଓ

Cetyl Myristoleate

In the journal *Pharmacological Research : the official journal of the Italian Pharmacological Society*. 2003 Jan;47(1):43-7.

KW Hunter, et al., studied...

"Verification of the Anti-Arthritis Properties of Cetyl Myristoleate Administered Orally and by Injection"

OBJECTIVE & METHODS: Cetyl myristoleate (CMO) was reported by Diehl and May [J Pharm Sci 83 (1994) 296] to block inflammation and prevent adjuvant-induced arthritis in rats. To verify this earlier work, we have synthesized pure CMO and tested its anti-arthritic properties in a collagen-induced arthritis model in DBA/1LacJ mice...

...CONCLUSION: Although the protective effect of CMO in collagen-induced arthritis observed in the present study was less dramatic than that reported earlier, our results confirm the anti-arthritic properties of pure CMO.

☙❧☙❧

Collagen Type II

In the journal *Arthritis Rheum.* 1998 Feb;41(2):290-7.

ML Barnett, et al., studied...

"Treatment of rheumatoid arthritis with oral type II collagen. Results of a multicenter, double-blind, placebo-controlled trial."

OBJECTIVE: Oral administration of cartilage-derived type II collagen (CII) has been shown to ameliorate arthritis in animal models of joint inflammation, and preliminary studies have suggested that this novel therapy is clinically beneficial and safe in patients with rheumatoid arthritis (RA). The present study was undertaken to test the safety and efficacy of 4 different dosages of orally administered CII in patients with RA.

METHODS: Two hundred seventy-four patients with active RA were enrolled at 6 different sites and randomized to receive placebo or 1 of 4 dosages (20, 100, 500, or 2,500 microg/day) of oral CII for 24 weeks. Efficacy parameters were assessed monthly. Cumulative response rates (percentage of patients meeting the criteria for response at any time during the study) were analyzed utilizing 3 sets of composite criteria: the Paulus criteria, the American College of Rheumatology criteria for improvement in RA, and a requirement for > or = 30% reduction in both swollen and tender joint counts...

...CONCLUSION: Positive effects were observed with CII at the lowest dosage tested, and the presence of serum antibodies to CII at baseline may predict response to therapy. No side effects were associated with this novel therapeutic agent. Further controlled studies are required to assess the efficacy of this treatment approach.

ཙཚཙཚ

Glucosamine & MSM

In the journal *Clinical Drug Investigation* 2004, vol. 24, no. 6, pp. 353-363(11)

PR Usha, et al., studied...

"Randomised, Double-Blind, Parallel, Placebo-Controlled Study of Oral Glucosamine, Methylsulfonylmethane and their Combination in Osteoarthritis"

Abstract:

Objective: Glucosamine, classified as a slow-acting drug in osteoarthritis (SADOA), is an efficacious chondroprotective agent. Methylsulfonylmethane (MSM), the isoxidised form of dimethylsulfoxide (DSMO), is an effective natural analgesic and anti-inflammatory agent. The aim of this study was to compare the efficacy and safety of oral glucosamine (Glu), methylsulfonylmethane (MSM), their combination and placebo in osteoarthritis of the knee.

Patients and design: A total of 118 patients of either sex with mild to moderate osteoarthritis were included in the study and randomised to receive either Glu 500mg, MSM 500mg, Glu and MSM or placebo capsules three times daily for 12 weeks. Patients were evaluated at 0 (before drug administration), 2, 4, 8 and 12 weeks post-treatment for efficacy and safety. The efficacy parameters studied were the pain index, the swelling index, visual analogue scale pain intensity, 15m walking time, the Lequesne index, and consumption of rescue medicine...

...Conclusion: Glu, MSM and their combination produced an analgesic and anti-inflammatory effect in osteoarthritis. Combination therapy showed better efficacy in reducing pain and swelling and in improving the functional ability of joints than the individual agents. All the treatments were well tolerated. The onset of analgesic and anti-inflammatory activity was found to be more rapid with the combination than with Glu. It can be concluded that the combination of MSM with Glu provides better and more rapid improvement in patients with osteoarthritis.

ME COMMENTS:

Dr. Usha's study shows that the combined effect of MSM and glucosamine is greater than the ingredients individually. Evidence from my clinical practice supports the concept that combining natural products, such as MSM, glucosamine, boswellia, cetyl myristoleate, collagen type II, have a synergistic effect on lowering muscle and joint pain. Similar to Dr. Usha's findings, the combined product has a great effect than the individual components.

ଓଡଓଡ

Glossary

ACE(Angiotensin Converting Enzyme) Inhibitors

Block an enzyme in the body that is responsible for causing the blood vessels to narrow. If the blood vessels are relaxed, your blood pressure is lowered and more oxygen-rich blood can reach your heart.

They lower the amount of salt and water in your body, which also helps to lower your blood pressure, i.e., Accupril® (quinapril), Aceon® (perindopril), Altace® (ramipril), Capoten® (captopril), Lotensin® (benazepril), Mavik® (trandolapril), Monopril® (fosinopril), Prinivil® (lisinopril), Univasc® (moexipril), Vasotec® (enalaprilat, enalapril), Zestril® (lisinopril).

ALA

Aminolevulinic acid - one of the oils in Omega3.

Aliphatic

Relating to or being an organic compound having an open chain structure.

Antioxidant

Any of various substances (as beta-carotene, vitamin C, and alpha-tocopherol) that inhibit oxidation or reactions promoted by oxygen and peroxides and that include many molecules held to protect the living body from the deleterious effects of free radicals.

Apoenzyme

A protein that forms an active enzyme system in combination with a coenzyme and determines the specificity of this system for a substrate.

Apoptotic / Apoptosis

Programmed cell death as signaled by the nuclei in normally functioning human and animal cells when age or state of cell health and condition dictates.

Cells that die by apoptosis do not usually elicit the inflammatory responses that are associated with necrosis, though the reasons are not clear.

Cancerous cells, however, are unable to experience the normal cell transduction or apoptosis-driven natural cell death process.

Atopic

A probably hereditary allergy characterized by symptoms (as asthma, hay fever, or hives) produced upon exposure especially by inhalation to the exciting environmental antigen.

Atopy

See atopic.

Beta Blockers

"Block" the effects of adrenaline on your body's beta receptors. This slows the nerve impulses that travel through the heart. As a result, your heart does not have to work as hard because it needs less blood and oxygen. The results are lowered heart rate and blood pressure. i.e. Betapace® (sotalol), Blocadren® (timolol), Brevibloc® (esmolol), Cartrol® (carteolol), Coreg® (carvedilol), Corgard® (nadolol), Inderal® (propranolol), Inderal-LA® (propranolol), Kerlone® (betaxolol), Levatol® (penbutolol), Lopressor® (metoprolol), Normodyne® (labetalol), Sectral® (acebutolol), Tenormin® (atenolol), Toprol-XL® (metoprolol), Trandate® (labetalol), Visken® (pindolol), Zebeta® (bisoprolol).

Bio-Identical

Hormones have the same chemical structure as hormones that are made by the human body. The term "bio-identical" does not indicate the source of the hormone, but rather indicates that the chemical structure of the replacement hormone is identical to that of the hormone naturally found in the human body. In order for a replacement hormone to fully replicate the function of hormones which were originally naturally produced and present in the human body, the chemical structure must exactly match the original. Bio-identical hormones are able to follow normal metabolic pathways so that essential active metabolites are formed in response to hormone replacement therapy.

Bonito Peptides

This natural supplement is composed of a purified mixture of 9 small peptides (proteins) derived from muscle of the fish bonito (a member of the tuna family) and is also free from heavy metals (e.g. lead, mercury, etc.), pesticides, and other contaminants.

Boswellia

This naturally occurring substance comes from the Boswellia serrata tree that grows in the dry hills of India. Preparations made from a purified extract of this resin are used to reduce inflammation associated with osteoarthritis and rheumatoid arthritis.

Unlike conventional NSAIDs, such as ibuprofen, Boswellia has no known side effects and doesn't seem to cause stomach irritation. It also may be effective for back pain and certain chronic intestinal disorders.

C. diff.

See Clostridium difficile.

C. difficile

See Clostridium difficile.

Calcium Channel Blockers

Slow the rate at which calcium passes into the heart muscle and into the vessel walls. This relaxes the vessels. The relaxed vessels let blood flow more easily through them, thereby lowering blood pressure. i.e. Adalat® (nifedipine), Calan® (verapamil), Cardene® (nicardipine), Cardizem® (diltiazem), Cardizem CD® (diltiazem), Cardizem SR®(diltiazem), Cartia® (diltiazem), Covera-HS® (verapamil), Dilacor XR® (diltiazem), Diltia XT® (diltiazem), DynaCirc® (isradipine), Isoptin® (verapamil), Lotrel® (amlodipine), Nimotop® (nimodipine), Norvasc® (amlodipine), Plendil® (felodipine), Procardia® (nifedipine), Procardia XL® (nifedipine), Sular® (nisoldipine), Tiamate® (diltiazem),Tiazac® (diltiazem), Vascor® (bepridil), Verelan® (verapamil).

CDAD

Clostridium difficile associated diarrhea.

Cetyl Myristoleate

Is derived from an environmentally friendly source, palmitic acid (a fatty acid in coconut and palm oils). Cetyl Myristoleate is a powerful anti-inflammatory agent. Additionally, it acts as a highly effective lubricant in joints, muscles and other tissues, allowing them to move more smoothly. It is also an immune system modulator which can be effectual against auto-immune conditions. All of these characteristics contribute to its ability to act as an analgesic by removing the source of pain (inflamed and irritated tissues) so that there is no pain impulse.

CHD

Coronary Heart Disease.

CHOLESTEROL

A waxy, fat-like substance manufactured in the liver and found in all tissues, it facilitates the transport and absorption of fatty acids. In foods, only animal products contain cholesterol. An excess of cholesterol in the bloodstream can contribute to the development of atherosclerosis.

CLOSTRIDIUM DIFFICILE

A spore-forming, gram-positive bacillus that produces exotoxins that are pathogenic to humans. C. difficile- associated disease (CDAD) ranges in severity from mild diarrhea to fulminant colitis and death. Antibiotic use is the primary risk factor for development of CDAD because it disrupts normal bowel flora and promotes C. difficile overgrowth.

CLOSTRIDIUM PERFRINGENS

An unhealthy bacteria commonly found in the human gastrointestinal tract.

COENZYME

An organic nonprotein molecule, frequently a phosphorylated derivative of a water soluble vitamin, that binds with the protein molecule (apoenzyme) to form the active enzyme (holoenzyme).

COENZYME Q10

A vital substance that assists in the oxidation of nutrients within cells to create energy. It is also highly efficient at protecting internal and external cell membranes against oxidation. All statin pharmaceuticals interfere with its production and thus require supplementation with CoQ10.

COLLAGEN TYPE II

Is a dietary supplement that supports skin, joint and connective tissue health. It is naturally rich in Hyaluronic Acid (HA) a Cartilage Matrix Glycoprotein (TMGP), powerful substances that help protect the cartilage from breakdown and promote cartilage synthesis.

Colonize

The formation of compact population groups of the same type of microorganism, as the colonies that develop when a bacterial cell begins reproducing.

Crestor® (rosuvastatin)

A chemically modified version of the statin found in nature.

CVD

Coronary Vessel Disease.

DHA

Docosahexaenoic Acid - one of the oils in Omega3.

Digestive Enzymes

Are proteins released from your salivary glands, stomach and small intestines, specially tailored to break down foods into nutrients that your body can readily digest.

Dysbiosis

An unhealthy balance of bacteria in the GI tract, involving an overgrowth of unhealthy organisms, including candida albicans and a variety of other harmful bacteria and parasites.

Endogenous

Relating to or produced by metabolic synthesis in the body.

Enzyme

A protein molecule produced by living organisms that catalyses chemical reactions of other substances without itself being destroyed or altered upon completion of the reactions.

EPA

Eicosapentaenoic Acid - one of the oils in Omega3.

Exogenous

Introduced from or produced outside the organism or system; specifically: not synthesized within the organism or system (i.e. Probiotics).

FERMENTATION

A process by which friendly bacteria obtain their energy by chemically breaking down sugars and proteins. The major breakdown products are the SCFA, such as acetic acid, butyric acid, proprionic acid. These SCFA are what bring about the beneficial effects of Probiotic bacteria. Metabolism of SCFA provides a source of energy for both humans and bacteria.

FOLIC ACID

A vitamin of the B complex that is required for normal production of red blood cells, that is used especially in the treatment of nutritional anemias, and that occurs especially in green leafy vegetables, liver, kidneys, dried beans, and mushrooms -- called also folacin, folate, Lactobacillus casei factor, pteroylglutamic acid, vitamin Bc, vitamin M. Scientific studies also shows that it has an effect on lowering blood pressure.

FOS

Fructooligosaccharide is a Prebiotic, a member of the family of Oligosaccharides, sugars linked together with undigestible bonds. The human body has no enzymes which can break the bonds and therefore cannot digest FOS. FOS passes untouched into the large intestines where they can be a food source for the beneficial bacteria who have the enzymes to break down the FOS bonds.

FREE RADICALS

Highly reactive molecules with an unsatisfied electron valence pair. Free radicals are produced in both normal and pathological processes. They are proven or suspected agents of tissue damage in a wide variety of circumstances including radiation, damage from environment chemicals, and aging. Natural and pharmacological prevention of free radical damage is being actively investigated.

FREEZE DRIED

To dry and preserve (as food, vaccines, or tissue) in a frozen state under high vacuum.

FRUCTOOLIGOSACCHARIDE

See FOS, Oligosaccharide & Prebiotic.

FXR

The Farneosid X Receptor (FXR) is a nuclear receptor that regulates gene expression in response to bile acids. It plays a central role in bile acids, cholesterol, and lipo protein metabolism.

GALACTOOLIGOSACCHARIDE

See GOS, Oligosaccharide & Prebiotic.

GLUCOSAMINE

An amino sugar normally formed in the body from glucose. It is the starting point for the synthesis of glycosaminoglycans (GAGs), including Hyaluronic Acid, a main constituent of joint fluid. Glucosamine supplementation can help support the thick gelatinous nature of the joint fluid, as well as proper functioning of joints, spinal disc, and other connective tissue.

GOS

Galactooligosaccharide is a Prebiotic, a member of the family of Oligosaccharides, sugars linked together with undigestible bonds. The human body has no enzymes which can break the bonds and therefore cannot digest GOS. GOS passes untouched into the large intestines where they can be a food source for the beneficial bacteria who have the enzymes to break down the GOS bonds. Also called Prebiotics.

GUGGULIPIDS

This natural ingredient is derived from the mixture of plant chemicals (ketonic steroids) from the gum resin of Commiphora mukul, called Guggulipid, and is an approved treatment of hyperlipidemia in India. It has been a mainstay of traditional Indian herbal medicine (Ayurveda) approaches in preventing high cholesterol and atherosclerosis. Clinical studies indicate it to be effective in the treatment of elevated cholesterol, elevated triglyceride levels and elevated LDL (bad cholesterol) levels. Studies have also shown that LDL oxidation, which is the main cause of plaque build in the arteries, can be prevented or at least decreased by the antioxidant activity of Guggul. Clinical studies on Guggul indicate that its hypolipidemic activity (decreasing cholesterol and other lipids) can be attributed to more than one mechanism. Three of the possible mechanisms include inhibition of cholesterol biosynthesis, enhancing the rate of excretion of cholesterol and promoting rapid degradation of cholesterol.

Guggul is typically manufactured in a standardized form that provides a fixed amount of Guggulipid, the presumed active ingredients

---

GUGGULIPIDS - CONTINUED

in Guggul. Guggul helps reduce high cholesterol, because it lowers harmful LDL (low-density lipoproteins) while elevating the beneficial HDL (high-density lipoproteins). Guggul also has anti-inflammatory activity and reduces the levels of C-reactive protein. It helps prevent blood platelet aggregation and breaks up blood clots. Thus Guggul can be used not only to lower bad cholesterol but can be used as a preventative against heart disease and stroke.

HIGH-DENSITY LIPOPROTEIN (HDL)

Also known as "good" cholesterol, HDLs are large, dense, protein-fat particles that circulate in the blood picking up already used and unused cholesterol and taking them back to the liver as part of a recycling process. Higher levels of HDLs are associated with a lower risk of cardiovascular disease because the cholesterol is cleared more readily from the blood.

HMG-COA REDUCTASE

Hydroxymethylglutaryl-CoA Reductase an enzyme in the pathway for the synthesis of cholesterol and CoQ10.

HMG-COA REDUCTASE INHIBITOR

Substances which inhibit the enzyme HMG-CoA Reductase thereby lowering cholesterol levels and inadvertently lowering CoQ10 levels. All statin pharmaceuticals are inhibitors of this enzyme and thereby bring about lowering of cholesterol levels and inadvertently lowering of CoQ10 levels.

HOLOENZYME

The complete enzyme complex composed of the protein portion (apoenzyme) and cofactor or coenzyme.

HYPERCHOLESTEROLEMIA

Excess cholesterol in the blood.

HYPERLIPIDEMIA

Increased cholesterol level.

HYPERTENSION

High blood pressure. Hypertension increases the risk of heart attack, stroke, and kidney failure because it adds to the workload of the heart, causing it to enlarge and, over time, to weaken; in addition, it may damage the walls of the arteries.

INOSITOL HEXONIACINATE

The form of Niacin that does not cause side effects, such as flushing and liver toxicity. Recent studies have shown that it lowers LDL cholesterol and raises HDL cholesterol.

LIPID (LIPIDS)

Fat-soluble substances derived from animal or vegetable cells by nonpolar solvents (e.g. ether); the term can include the following types of materials: fatty acids, glycerides, phospholipids, alcohols and waxes.

LIPITOR® (ATORVASTATIN)

A chemically modified version of the statin found in nature.

LIPOPROTEINS (LIPOPROTEIN)

Molecules composed of lipids and proteins that carry fats and cholesterol through the bloodstream.

LOVASTATIN

Generic for Merck's brand Mevacor, it is the naturally occurring statin Monacolin-K.

LOW-DENSITY LIPOPROTEIN (LDL)

Also known as "bad" cholesterol, LDLs are large, dense, protein-fat particles composed of a moderate proportion of protein and a high proportion of cholesterol. Higher levels of LDLs are associated with a greater risk of cardiovascular disease.

LYOPHILIZE

Freeze-dried.

MANNANOLIGOSACCHARIDES

See MOS, Oligosaccharides & Prebiotics.

Mevacor

Merck's brand name for Monacolin-K (generic name Lovastatin).

Mixed Tocopherols

Any of several fat-soluble vitamins that are chemically tocopherols or tocotrienols, are essential in the nutrition of various vertebrates in which their absence is associated with infertility, degenerative changes in muscle, or vascular abnormalities, are found especially in wheat germ, vegetable oils, egg yolk, and green leafy vegetables or are made synthetically, and are used chiefly in animal feeds and as antioxidants; especially : Alpha-Tocopherol.

Monacolin-K

One of the nine naturally occurring substances found in Red Yeast Rice which inhibits HMG-CoA Reductase activity.

Monacolins

Natural substances found in Red Yeast Rice which interfere with the pathway of HMG-CoA reductase. (i.e. Monacolin-K, Monacolins-I,II,III,IV,V,VI, Dihydromonacolin.)

Monascus

A type of yeast added to red rice in order to produce the fermented product Red Yeast Rice.

MOS

Mannanoligosaccharide is a Prebiotic, a member of the family of Oligosaccharides, that binds potentially harmful bacteria in the gut and allows beneficial bacteria to dominate; also assists immune function.

MSM (Methyl Sulfonyl Methane) Complex

This naturally occurring sulfur compound has a vitamin like normalizing influence on body functions. It helps to regulate pro-inflammatory enzymes to reduce pain and swelling associated with connective tissue dysfunction.

Natural

Occurs in nature. Although it occurs in nature - may not be natural to a certain species.

Natural Pharmaceuticals

Substances found in nature that are digestible as food sources, that have not been altered from their original form but have been made into tablet or capsule form.

Niacin

Member of the water soluble B vitamin group (vitamin B3), used in the production of fatty acids, steroids and cholesterol, deficiency is known as pellagra. Has cholesterol-lowering and vasodilating properties. It also has been shown to cause flushing (see Inositol Hexoniacinate).

Non-Colonize

Does not colonize (see colonize).

Non-Pathogenic

Not capable of causing disease.

Octacosanol

See Policosanol.

Oligosaccharide

Is the "family name" of a category of small, digested in the colon (non-digestible in the intestine) sugars that are food for the friendly bacteria. [Oligo = small & Saccharide = sugar]

Some examples, Frutooligosaccharide (FOS), Mannan-oligosaccharides (MOS) & Galactooligosaccharides (GOS).

Omega3

Being or composed of polyunsaturated fatty acids which are found especially in fish (as tuna and salmon), fish oils, green leafy vegetables, and some vegetable oils. Has been shown to lower cholesterol and blood pressure levels.

Pathogenic

Capable of causing disease.

Peptide

A compound of two or more amino acids (the building blocks of all protein molecules).

PHYTO

Derived from plants.

PHYTOCHEMICALS

Chemicals derived from plants.

PHYTOSTANOLS

See sterols and stanols. Phyto means derived from plants.

PHYTOSTEROLS

See sterols and stanols. Phyto means derived from plants.

POLICOSANOL

Is the generic term used for a mixture of long chain fatty alcohols, derived chiefly from the waxy coating of sugar cane and used as a dietary supplement to lower cholesterol levels.

Policosanol belongs to a family of wax-like phytochemicals prevalent throughout nature. This substance is used in the dietary supplement industry sourced from several foods that include: sugar cane, rice bran, beeswax, broccoli, spinach, alfalfa and oats.

Sugar cane derived Policosanol is a new face on the cholesterol scene in the United States but is a popular hypocholesterolemic in other countries. The main Policosanol form in sugar cane is Octacosanol, a long-chain fatty alcohol found in the waxy film that covers the leaves and fruit of the plants that contain it.

Triacontanol & Octacosanol are the main components of the Policosanol complex followed by Tetracosanol and Hexacosanol all which are found naturally within Octacosanol.

PREBIOTICS

Are non-digestible food ingredients that beneficially affect the host by selectively stimulating the growth of one or a limited number of bacteria in the colon. The colonic bacteria to be stimulated are Bifidobacterium and/or Lactobacilli.

The non-digestible character of Prebiotics is a feature shared with dietary fibre but their physiological functions are often different. Thus, the Prebiotics are very selective in their growth stimulation and at the same time they suppress many pathogenic bacteria present in the microbiota because they can only use the Prebiotic ingredient for growth to a limited extent or not at all. Thus, the Prebiotic principle is based on selective stimulation of those colonic microorganisms able to break down (hydrolyse) the Prebiotics to carbohydrate monomers (simple carbohydrates) and use those for growth.

PREBIOTICS - CONTINUED

Two principal types commonly used are: 1. Mannanoligosaccharides (MOS) that bind potentially harmful bacteria in the gut and allow beneficial bugs to dominate; also assists immune function. 2. Fructooligosaccharides (FOS) that deliver fructans into the fore gut to 'feed' the acid producing bacteria (the families of Lactobacillus and Bifidobacterium).

Other useful prebiotics include: Galactooligosaccharides, Xylitol (Xyllooligosaccharides), Manitol, Sorbitol, Arabinogalatose, etc.

PREVACHOL® (PRADASTATIN)

A chemically modified version of the statin found in nature.

PROBIOTICS

Probiotics are living microorganisms (bacterial or yeast) which upon ingestion in certain numbers exert health benefits beyond inherent basic nutrition. Probiotic means "for life" (as opposed to antibiotic which means "anti life").

All known Probiotic bacteria belong to the group called lactic acid bacteria, which in this context includes the species Lactococcus, Lactobacillus, Streptococcus, Leuconostoc, Pediococcus, Bifidobacterium and Enterococcus.

To be a successful Probiotic, the bacteria must fulfil the following criteria:

Be safe (e.g. of human origin and non-pathogenic)

Be resistant to technologic processes and exert minimal sensory influence on the Probiotic food.

Be resistant to passage through the gastrointestinal tract (gastric acidity and bile acids).

Adhere to the gut epithelial tissue and possess growth capability.

Provide health benefits.

Red Yeast Rice

Has been used in China for centuries as both a food and as a medicinal substance. Red Yeast Rice is the fermented product of rice on which red yeast (Monascus Purpureus) has been grown. In Chinese medicine, Red Yeast Rice is used to promote blood circulation, soothe upset stomach, and invigorate the function of the spleen, a body organ that destroys old blood cells and filters foreign substances. In addition, this dietary supplement has been used traditionally for bruised muscles, hangovers, indigestion, and colic in infants.

The use of Red Yeast Rice in China was first documented in the Tang Dynasty in 800 AD. It has been used to make rice wine, as a food preservative for maintaining the color and taste of fish and meat, and for its medicinal properties.

Rhabdomyolysis

The destruction or degeneration of skeletal muscle tissue (as from traumatic injury, excessive exertion, or stroke) that is accompanied by the release of muscle cell contents (as myoglobin and potassium) into the bloodstream resulting in hypovolemia, hyperkalemia, and sometimes acute renal failure.

Saccromyces Boullardii

A non pathogenic Friendly Yeast (Probiotic) widely prescribed in a lyophilized form, used in adults and children as a biotherapeutic agent. Controlled clinical trials have demonstrated the efficacy of Saccromyces Boullardii for preventing or treating several intestinal disorders including AAD (Antibiotic Associated Diarrhea), recurrent Clostridium Difficile Disease, acute diarrhea in children and adults, travelers' diarrhea, diarrhea in tube fed patients, AIDS related diarrhea and relapses of Chrones Disease and Ulcerative Cholitis.

Short Chain Fatty Acids (SCFA)

Compounds produced by beneficial bacteria as a result of consuming fibers like FOS. SCFAs are responsible for many of the desirable effects of FOS, including reduction in future putrfactive substances and cholesterol lowering. Promotes growth of ephithelial cells that line the colon. It acts like glue on the intestinal lining to prevent pathological bacteria from adhering to the surface walls.

SHR

Albino rats bred from a male with mild hypertension, mated with a female with high blood pressure. Brother X, sister mating with continued selection for high blood pressure.

STATINS (STATIN)

A class of drugs that lower cholesterol.

STEROL

Any of the solid steroid alcohols (as cholesterol) widely distributed in animal and plant lipids.

STEROLS AND STANOLS

Sterols and Stanols represent a group of compounds that are an essential constituent of cell membranes in animals and plants. Cholesterol is actually a sterol of human cells, whereas phytosterols are produced by plants (also called phytosterols and phytostanols). The most common plant sterols are sitosterol, campesterol, and stigmasterol. Plant sterols, although structurally similar to cholesterol, are not synthesized by the human body and are very poorly absorbed. The specific plant sterols that are currently incorporated into foods and supplements are extracted from soybean oil. The plant sterols, currently incorporated into foods, are esterified to unsaturated fatty acids (creating sterol esters) to increase lipid solubility, thus allowing maximal incorporation into a limited amount of fat. Some plant sterols currently available are saturated, to form the stanol derivatives, which are also effective at lowering cholesterol.

STEVIA

Is an herb with incredible sweetening power. Its ability to sweeten is rated between 70 to 400 times that of white sugar. It is completely natural in its biochemical profile. Unlike other natural sweetening agents, it is completely calorie free, never initiates a rise in blood sugar, does not provide food for microorganisms like bacteria and yeast, and has been shown to lower blood pressure.

SYMBIOSIS

A type of organism-organism interaction where one organism lives in intimate association with another.

SYNBIOTICS

The combining of Prebiotics with Probiotics, i.e. Probiotics + MOS, Probiotics + FOS.

SYNERGISTIC

"Used esp. of drugs or muscles that work together so the total effect is greater than the sum of the two (or more)".

TEN

Total Enteral Nutrition.

TOCOPHEROLS

Functions as an antioxidant, binds oxygen free radicals that can cause tissue damage, may also play a protective role in the coronary arteries from the damaging effects of cholesterol.

TRAVELER'S DIARRHEA

Diarrhea suffered by tourists when traveling to foreign parts.

TRIACONTANOL

See Policosanol.

TRIGLYCERIDE (TRIGLYCERIDES)

The main form of fat found in foods and the human body. Containing three fatty acids and one unit of glycerol, triglycerides are stored in adipose cells in the body, which, when broken down, release fatty acids into the blood. Triglycerides are fat storage molecules and are the major lipid component of the diet.

TROPHIC

Promoting cellular growth, differentiation, and survival.

VITAMIN B3

Also known as Niacin.

VITAMINS

Any of various organic substances that are essential in minute quantities to the nutrition of most animals and some plants, act especially as coenzymes and precursors of coenzymes in the regulation of metabolic processes but do not provide energy or serve as building units, and are present in natural foodstuffs or are sometimes produced within the body.

ZOCOR® (SIMVASTATIN)

A chemically modified version of the statin found in nature.

APPENDIX A
Know Your Cholesterol Levels

Total Cholesterol

Desirable	Less than 200 mg/dL
Borderline high risk	200–239 mg/dL
High risk	240 mg/dL and over

LDL Cholesterol Level - The lower the better
(Low Density Lipoproteins - bad cholesterol)

Less than 100 mg/dL	Optimal
100 to 129 mg/dL	Near Optimal/ Above Optimal
130 to 159 mg/dL	Borderline High
160 to 189 mg/dL	High
190 mg/dL and above	Very High

HDL Cholesterol Levels - The higher the better
(High Density Lipoproteins - good cholesterol)

average man	40 to 50 mg/dL
average woman	50 to 60 mg/dL

Triglyceride Level

Triglyceride Level	Classification
Less than 150 mg/dL	Normal
150–199 mg/dL	Borderline-high
200–499 mg/dL	High
500 mg/dL or higher	Very high

APPENDIX B

Know Your Blood Pressure Level

Blood pressure is measured in millimeters of mercury (mm Hg). The classifications in the table below are for people who are not taking blood pressure-lowering drugs and are not acutely ill.

When a person's systolic and diastolic pressures fall into different categories, the higher category is used to classify the blood pressure status.

Classification of blood pressure for adults age 18 years and older

Category	Systolic (mm Hg) upper #		Diastolic (mm Hg) lower #
Normal	less than 120	and	less than 80
Prehypertension	120-139	or	80-89
Stage 1 Hypertension	140-159	or	90-99
Stage 2 Hypertension	160 or higher	or	100 or higher

(From the Seventh Report of the Joint National Committee on Detection, Evaluation, and Treatment of High Blood Pressure)

APPENDIX C

Excerpts from...

Testimony Before the House Government Reform Committee

By David Heber, M.D., Ph.D., FACP, FACN July 25, 2002

I am a Professor of Medicine and Public Health and the Founding Director of the UCLA Center for Human Nutrition and the Division of Clinical Nutrition at the David Geffen School of Medicine at UCLA with federal funding for centers and training of physicians and scientists from three NIH Institutes including the National Cancer Institute, the National Institute of Diabetes, Digestive and Kidney Diseases, and the Office of Dietary Supplements Research in cooperation with the National Center for Complementary and Alternative Medicine. Over the past 20 years, I have participated in and witnessed a revolutionary expansion of our knowledge of nutrition science and the benefits of fruits, vegetables and dietary supplements including botanical dietary supplements. When I attended medical school almost 30 years ago, I was taught that you get all the vitamins you need by eating the basic four food groups. Today, we know that is not true and that there is a great deal of evidence suggesting that four basic vitamins including multivitamins with folic acid, vitamin E, vitamin C and calcium can benefit all Americans by reducing the risk of chronic diseases. Unfortunately, scientific breakthroughs and insights such as these are not being translated into health benefits for our population as the jurisdiction for the regulation of nutrition information is divided among several different agencies with different primary missions including the USDA, the NIH, the CDC, the FDA, and the FTC. The discovery of hybrid corn in 1938 contributed to national security by helping this nation win World War II, and a grain surplus continues to insure our national security. However, 70% of that grain is fed to domesticated animals for dairy and meat production. Refined sugars such as high fructose corn syrup (the cola sweetener) and vegetable oils increase hidden calories in popular snack foods marketed to our children. In fact, it is estimated that 1/3 of all Americans get 47% of their calories from so-called junk foods...

...Botanical dietary supplements are at the growing edge of nutrition science, and represent the restoration of even greater diversity than can be accomplished with increased servings of fruits and vegetables. Spices such as garlic and curcumin have been known since ancient times to have health benefits. **At UCLA, I directed the first U.S. clinical trial showing that Chinese Red Yeast Rice can be as effective as prescription drugs for lowering cholesterol.** This ancient spice is a distant relative of the red spice on Peking Duck and Pork Spare Ribs available at your local Chinese restaurant. The difference between that spice and the traditional spice is that modern spice is made by liquid fermentation and does not have the same phytochemicals contained in yeast fermented by the traditional Chinese method on a bed of premium rice. Red yeast rice made this way is a traditional food consumed throughout Asia for its food and medicinal value for over a thousand years with the first written documentation in 800 A.D. The fungus Monascus isolated from Red yeast rice first became known in Western society through the work of Dutch scientists who noted its use by local populations in Java as reported by Van Tieghem et al. in 1884. A species isolated from red Koji or Honqu (as red rice yeast is known in East Asia) was named Monascus Purpureus Went in 1895 recognizing the purple coloration. Today there are more than 30 Monascus strains on deposit with the American Type Culture Collection (Bethesda, MD) and it was declared a food product by the USDA in the 1920's.

There are 57 million Americans with high cholesterol and only 13 million take prescription drugs for cholesterol lowering. Mevacor at 20 mg to 40 mg per day has been shown to reduce heart disease deaths and heart attacks by 30% over 5 years in individuals with modestly high cholesterol levels. I suspect that Chinese Red Yeast Rice would have the same public health benefit at lower cost,...

...It is my view that we have the finest government in the world, the finest agriculture in the world and the finest medical research and drug development institutions in the world. However, these complex institutions are not working in concert to optimize health in this country. **Hippocrates said in 500 BC "let food be your medicine and let your medicine be food." Our 21st Century science has brought us full circle to realize that it is no accident that 2/3 of our drugs are derived from plants or that vitamin deficiency diseases only became evident when and where mankind doesn't have a varied intake of plant products.** A single orange has 170% of the recommended dietary allowance of vitamin C but it also has in its skin a fatty substance the citrus fruits developed to fight off fungi (called limonoids) which also happen to inhibit cancer cell growth. Drugs have their place and so do botanical dietary supplements....

...The entire testimony can be found at:

http://www.cancercurecoalition.org/articles/nutritionandcancer.html

APPENDIX D

Excerpts from...

In the *Gastroenterology Clinics of North America*, Volume 34 • Number 3 • September 2005, pages 413-436.

Stig Bengmark, MD, PhD studied...

"Bioecologic Control of the Gastrointestinal Tract: The Role of Flora and Supplemented Probiotics and Synbiotics"

...The World Health Organization estimates that 46% of global disease burden and 59% of global mortality are due to chronic disease; 35 million individuals die each year from chronic diseases, and this statistic has been increasing steadily. The increase, which seems to have its beginning at the time of the Industrial Revolution (e.g., the mid-1850s), was relatively slow during the first 100 years, but during recent decades the increase in morbidity and mortality has obtained epidemic proportions. Circumstantial evidence supports an association of chronic disease with the transition from natural unprocessed foods to processed and often calorie-condensed foods. The correlation between increases in chronic diseases and reduction in intake of plant fibers and plant antioxidants with increase in consumption of refined sugars is obvious; the individual consumption of sugar has increased from about 1 lb/person/y in 1850 to about 100 lb/person/y in 2000...

...FOOD CONNECTION

The modern Western lifestyle is characterized not only by significant alterations in food consumption. Stress; lack of physical exercise; use of alcohol, tobacco, and pharmaceuticals, and increasing exposure to environmental chemicals also seem to contribute to the burden of chronic disease in Western society. Foods that are consumed—refined and calorie-condensed food products—contain large amounts of saturated and trans fatty acids, sugar and starch, and bioactive peptides such as gluten and are low in omega-3 polyunsaturated fatty acids, plant antioxidants, and health-promoting plant fibers and bacteria. Common to most of the above-mentioned food ingredients is that they affect the function of the innate immune system, the inflammatory response, and the individual's resistance to disease. Plant fibers, antioxidants, and, to some extent, polyunsaturated fatty acids enforce the resistance to disease, whereas saturated and trans fatty acids, sugar and starch, peptides such as gluten, and many chemicals and pharmaceuticals, including antibiotics, suppress the resistance to disease. Consequently, most patients with chronic disease have increased acute and chronic phase response, increased inflammation/superinflammation, and metabolic syndrome. Saturated fat and trans fatty acids induce significant alterations in the immune response; inhibit the macrophage functions; stimulate the Th2 response relative to the Th1 response; and increase the risk of getting chronic diseases, such as diabetes, certain cancers, and rheumatoid arthritis. Antibiotics result in suppression of the various macrophage functions, including chemiluminescence response, chemotactic motility, bactericidal and cytostatic ability, and lymphocyte proliferation.

The links between chronic diseases of the gastrointestinal tract, especially inflammatory bowel disease (IBD) and irritable bowel syndrome (IBS), and chronic phase response and metabolic syndrome have not been studied to the extent they should....

...Early humans did not consume grains or cow's milk, and most of the food they ate was vigorously fermented, as it was commonly stored in the soil for days, weeks, and months. Early humans consumed considerably less salt, fat, and sugar, but consumed about twice as much minerals, 10 times more plant fibers, greater than 20 times more antioxidants, greater than 50 times more omega-3 fatty acids, and billions of times more live bacteria.

...YOGURT AS CARRIER OF PROBIOTICS AND SYNBIOTICS

Cow's milk is not an ideal carrier of probiotics, especially for specific clinical use. In addition to its proposed role as risk factor for chronic diseases, concerns with cow's milk include the following:

1. Cow's milk is a poor carrier of bioactive fiber-fermenting probiotics because, in sharp contrast to breast milk, it contains no fibers or fiber-like molecules (only elephant milk contains as much as human milk). The complex fucosylated oligosaccharides in human milk, with structural similarities to immunomodulating cell surface glycoconjugates, protect breast-fed infants against infection and inflammation. These oligosaccharides most likely also serve as prebiotics, provide key nutrients to breast-fed infants, and

stimulate growth of the nonpathogenic health-supporting gut microflora.

2. Cow's milk is known to release inflammatory mediators; induce inflammation; induce leakage of molecules, such as albumin and hyaluronan; increase intestinal permeability; and cause translocation and leaky gut.

3. Cow's milk is known to be rich in free polyunsaturated fatty acids. It was shown that presence of polyunsaturated fatty acids, even in lower concentrations than provided in fermented dairy products such as yogurt, cause Lactobacillus to lose their ability to adhere to mucous membranes and to grow, supporting that dairy products are not ideal as carriers of probiotics.

Supplementing with yogurt bacteria or similar bacteria yields small or no clinical benefits....

...SUMMARY

Prebiotic, probiotic, and synbiotic treatment is still in its infancy. Although remarkable effects have been observed, extensive studies are necessary to understand the many mechanisms behind the observed effects. Compared with acute conditions, chronic diseases seem much more resistant to attempts to affect the course by modification of microbiota....

...Almost 100 years have passed since Metchnikoff suggested health benefits from external health-promoting bacteria and almost 50 years since Eiseman et al reported successful treatment with fecal enemas in antibiotic-associated pseudomembranous enterocolitis. Clinicians since have not administered the inheritance well....

ME COMMENTS:

Nature has given us the answer to so many chronic conditions while our scientists keep looking for more and more esoteric cures. Let us hope and pray that today's clinician will administer the inheritance of Dr. Metchnikoff and Eiseman better in the future than they have in the past.

APPENDIX E

Dr. Eisenstein's Treatment Protocols

for details and dosages go to

www.unlockingnaturespharmacy.com
www.homefirst.com

General Principles That Should Apply to All Persons

1) Reduce/eliminate refined carbohydrates
2) Increase exercise
3) Stop smoking

AAD (Antibiotic Associated Diarrhea)

Saccharomyces Boulardii

FOS

Probiotics + FOS

AD (Atopic Dermatitis)

Probiotics + FOS

Saccharomyces Boulardii

Digestive Enzymes

CHOLESTEROL

Primary Importance

Cholesterol Health™

Probiotics + FOS

Secondary Importance

Inositol Hexaniacinate , Mixed Tocopherols, Omega 3, CoQ10, FOS

Dr. Eisenstein's Treatment Protocols - Continued

CONSTIPATION

FOS Capsules

HEARTBURN, ACID REFLUX/GERD

Digestive Enzymes

HYPERTENSION

(Primary Importance)

Blood Pressure Support™

Probiotics + FOS

(Secondary Importance)

Omega 3, Co-Q10, FOS, Blood Pressure Support Plus™

IBD (Irritable Bowel Syndrome)

Probiotics + FOS

Saccharomyces Boulardii

Digestive Enzymes

INFECTION (No antibiotics prescribed)

Probiotics + MOS

Saccharomyces Boulardii

MENOPAUSAL SYMPTOMS

Natural Progesterone Cream

Probiotics + FOS

Dr. Eisenstein's Treatment Protocols - Continued

MUSCLE & JOINT PAIN

All Flex®

PREGNANCY

Probiotics + FOS

Prenatal Vitamins with digestive enzymes

PROSTATE HEALTH

Prostate Health™

Probiotics + FOS

Natural Progesterone Cream - Men

ભ્ઋભ્ઋ

Recommended Reading

Bacteria for Breakfast - "Probiotics for Good Health," by Dr. Kelly Karpa, Trafford Publishing, Victoria, BC, Canada 2003.

Statin Drugs Side Effects "and the Misguided War on Cholesterol" by Duane Graveline, M.D., 2005 www.SpaceDoc.net

Unavoidably Dangerous Medical Hazards of Synthetic HRT, by Mayer Eisenstein, MD, JD, MPH, 2003, CMI Press, Chapter 5, "Natural Progesterone Cream" Pages 127 - 140. Appendix B - "Natural Progesterone Cream for Men" Pages 165-174.

Safer Medicine Towards Clinical Scientific Evidence Based Medicine, by Mayer Eisenstein, MD, JD, MPH, CMI Press 2000, Chapter VI, Antibiotics pages 159-168 & Chapter XII Low Carbohydrate Lifestyle, pages 271-286.

www.homefirst.com

www.unlockingnaturespharmacy.com

www.thedoctorandthepharmacist.com

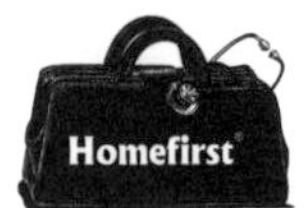

About Homefirst®

www.homefirst.com

Homefirst® Health Services provides a full range of services in family health care in the greater Chicago metropolitan area with four medical centers. Our medical staff of doctors and nurses, dedicate themselves to providing the highest quality of health care standards while maintaining personalized care for each patient and family. We encourage patient involvement in the many decisions made regarding their health care.

Since 1973 the Homefirst® doctors have been providing homebirth, pediatrics and adult care. They have delivered over 15,000 babies at home with less than 5% cesarean section rate and minimal use of drugs and intervention. **Now they are applying the same principles of minimal pharmaceuticals to adult medicine with emphasis on natural substitutes to control high blood pressure, high cholesterol, muscle and joint pain and other medical conditions.**

The Homefirst® doctors promote an integrative evidence based approach to managing illness. The majority of health problems are resolved by our medical staff. When necessary, we provide referrals to a wide variety of consultants which include practitioners in alternative approaches to medicine as well as conventional medical specialists.

Homefirst® offers complimentary seminars featuring Dr. Mayer Eisenstein, on cholesterol, blood pressure, and probiotics, homebirth, vaccines and a natural pharmaceutical seminar with Mark Mandel, compounding pharmacist.

ഁശ്ശ

About The Author

MAYER EISENSTEIN, MD, JD, MPH

Medical Director Homefirst® Health Services
Assistant Medical Director AMI *(Alternative Medicine Integration)*

Dr. Mayer Eisenstein is a graduate of the University of Illinois Medical School, the Medical College of Wisconsin School of Public Health, and the John Marshall Law School. In his 33 years in medicine, he and his practice have cared for over 75,000 parents, grandparents and children.

He is Board Certified by the National Board of Medical Examiners, American Board of Public Health and Preventive Medicine, and the American Board of Quality Assurance and Utilization Review Physicians. He is a recipient of the Howard Fellowship, Health Professional Scholarship, University of Illinois School of Medicine Scholarship, and is a member of the Illinois Bar.

He is the author of: *Give Birth at Home With The Home Birth Advantage*; *Safer Medicine, Don't Vaccinate Before You Educate; and Unavoidably Dangerous - Medical Hazards of HRT.* His medical film "Primum Non Nocere" (Above All Do No Harm), a documentary on home birth, was an award winner at the Chicago Film Festival in 1987.

Some of his guest appearances include: the "Phil Donahue Show", "Milt Rosenberg Show", "Today in Chicago", "Ask the Expert", "Daybreak", "Oprah Winfrey Show", "Ed Schwartz Radio Show", "Hannity and Colmes" on Mandatory Immunizations. "WMAQ TV news 'Unnecessary Hysterectomy'", "Chicago Fox TV News - 'Immunizations - Are They Necessary?'", CBC Newsworld Canada - "Are Mass Immunizations Necessary?".

Since 1987, his weekly radio show "The Doctor & The Pharmacist", has aired in the Chicagoland area. In the live call-in format, all listeners comments, questions or medical experiences are welcome by Dr. Eisenstein along with Mark Mandel, compounding pharmacist.

Dr. Eisenstein's latest seminar *"Saturdays with Dr. Eisenstein"* is devoted to two of the serious medical problems in our society, high blood pressure and high cholesterol. Scientific studies have shown that treating these conditions early can increase life expectancy and lower the incidence of stroke and heart disease. Dr. Eisenstein will discuss natural formulations which can help you avoid the need for pharmaceutical drugs in virtually all cases.

Dr. Eisenstein's philosophy comes from his years in medicine, law and Public Health, combined with his years as a husband, father, and grandfather.